BLOG TO BOOK

2.0

RICHARD NIKOLEY
Free the Animal

How to lose weight and fat on the Paleo diet

Table of Contents

I.

Introduction

The Popularity of the "Primitive Diet"

If you've been watching or reading the news over the past couple of years, you may have noticed references to bizarre new terms: the Paleo diet, the Caveman diet, and the Evolutionary diet. Perhaps you've seen variations on these themes that that seem familiar.

What does the popularity of these "primitive" diets mean?

It means a couple of things. The most important thing it means is that *something is wrong.* You'd think we were in the Golden Age of sound, peer-reviewed medical, diet, and nutrition advice; it's hard to go a day without seeing some news piece telling us what to eat and how to exercise. But for the past 30–40 years people in the United States have generally become fatter, weaker, and less healthy. They have become less virile as males, less sexually attractive as females.

Pictures of folks from decades past show that they were all pretty lean. Do you imagine they may have been starving? I don't think so. Instead, might it be possible that the advice we've been given over the last four decades—advice couched as "Dietary Guidelines for All Americans"—has been completely wrong?

Have you ever wondered why one guy can "eat like a horse," stay perfectly lean, and live to age 90, while one girl "eats like a bird," seems to always be hungry and miserable, and yet carries around 50 pounds of fat that would only be necessary if she were about to go into hibernation like a bear for a few months? You can reverse the gender, because examples abound.

I think women and men should be hot and enjoy that status for as long as possible. Isn't desiring each other what most fundamentally advances the human species? I think everyone should have the opportunity to jump, climb, run, and play—to be *active like the animals we are* for as long as nature allows. I think people should be aware of the adverse health effects of eating processed food composed of grains, refined sugar, and vegetable/seed oils, and equally aware of the fact that there's a different way to eat that can prevent and even cure the diseases of civilization.

A common objection to my pointing to governmental and institutional dietary guidelines as being behind the obesity epidemic is this: maybe it's that Americans aren't actually following the "Dietary Advice for all Americans," as proclaimed from on high. They're eating whatever they want, primarily junk food.

My answer is that Americans, in large measure, eat what's available at their local supermarkets, and that it's the multinational "food" conglomerates who have generally followed the dietary guidelines, selling their wares through clever marketing. Everything is fortified or "low in fat." Those guidelines have presented a marvelous profit opportunity for companies that produce cheap, attractive, and tasty products. To access these "food" items, humans have only to place them in a shopping cart and later apply some pressure to the glue that seals the flaps of the boxes together.

Eat and repeat.

I'm not a doctor. Not a dietitian. Not a medical or health researcher. I have a degree in business administration, and my first few jobs after college revolved around helping to make ships in the American and French navies run right. Later, in 1992, I became an entrepreneur. I failed, failed again, and eventually got a few things right and built a great company. Unfortunately, that was when nature started taking hold of me in adverse ways, in terms of body composition and health.

At some point in the mid 2000s, I found myself fat, generally disgusting, and unhealthy on many levels.

And then I fixed it. I blogged about my journey on Free the Animal (freetheanimal.com), eventually building a following that amounts to over 100,000 visits and over 200,000 page views per month. I have acquired many readers and correspondents who *are* medical doctors, researchers and other professional health practitioners. I've been interviewed for magazine articles, radio shows and various podcasts. I've been invited to speak at a few conferences.

What I have to say is working for people. It has worked for me and it has worked for thousands who comment on my blog regularly, providing their own unsolicited testimonials. I have a story to tell and a few words of advice, if you want to take them in.

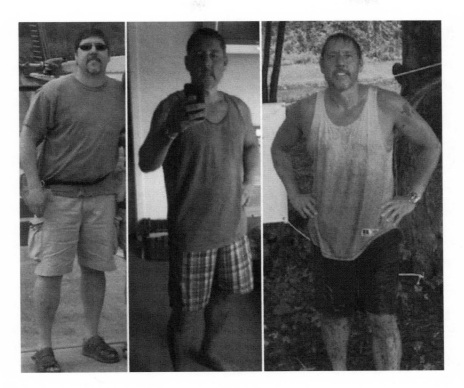

Disclaimer:

This e-book features weight-loss techniques that may not be suitable for everyone. You should always consult with a qualified medical practitioner before starting any weight-loss program, or if you have any concerns about your health. This e-book is not tailored to individual requirements or needs and its contents are solely for general information purposes. Nothing in it should be taken as professional or medical advice or diagnosis. The activities detailed in this e-book should not be used as a substitute for any treatment or medication prescribed or recommended to you by a medical practitioner. The author and the publishers do not accept any responsibility for any adverse effects that may occur as a result of the use of the suggestions or information herein. If you feel that you are experiencing adverse effects after embarking on any weight-loss program, including the type described in this e-book, it is imperative that you seek medical advice. Results may vary from individual to individual.

Note To Readers:

For those reading this book in print or on a device that's not web-enabled, please be aware that the author makes significant use of in-line hyperlinks to articles and references on the web, as well as lists of additional resources on the web. For those of you without the capability to click over, the author has made available a web page with all of the links in one place, chapter by chapter. Just go there on your computer to investigate them all, or only the ones you wish.

http://freetheanimal.com/book2-links

Become a Hyperink reader. Get a special surprise.

Like the book? Support our author and leave a comment!

II.

The Paleo, Primal, Ancestral Lifestyle

Escape From the Processed Food Culture The Paleo Way

Drawing on evolutionary logic, scientific research, and most importantly, my personal experience, I have come to the firm conclusion that mainstream dietary advice is not only wrong, it is maiming and killing those who follow it. In addition to devastating families, the Standard American Diet (SAD) is imposing tremendous costs that will ultimately be covered by healthier people—and the medical and drug industries are reaping the profits.

Processed Food Culture

Four years ago, I was on my way to becoming a victim of the SAD. Like many other Americans, my diet consisted largely of grain, sugar, and modern vegetable-oil based processed foods and fast foods. I made poor choices at restaurants and other eateries, consuming a lot of pizza, deep fried foods, and enormous portion sizes. When I was trying to eat well, I ate bread, cereal, rice, and corn products that were packaged as "healthy" choices.

I didn't see anything particularly wrong with my diet. I cooked what I thought was good, wholesome food at home a few times per week. Everyone else seemed to be eating the same stuff, and it didn't occur to me to question conventional wisdom. I was unaware that the processed and fast food culture is the reason so many Americans face obesity and ill health in modern times.

I was 160 pounds when I graduated high school. Normal adult weight at my height would probably be around 170. In 2007, *I tipped the scale at about 240 pounds.* This, after embarking on a religious daily walking regimen with my dog for five to six years, three to four miles per day, and about 6,000 miles total. I'd begun my routine when I weighed about 210 pounds, 30 less than where I topped out. I decided it's true that "insanity is doing the same thing over and over, expecting a different result." I had no excuse: it was time to start doing something differently.

The Beginning Of A New Lifestyle

In May of 2007, I had blood pressure soaring into the 160/100 range at virtually every check. I did some research on the Internet and found that heavy weight training can be effective in natural blood pressure regulation without drugs, so I hit the gym. It worked: my blood pressure began coming down immediately.

I wrote about my experience on my blog, **Free the Animal**. A commenter told me my new exercise routine sounded like professor Arthur De Vany's "power law training." Art, one of the original proponents of the Evolutionary Fitness lifestyle, recommends intense, brief exercise, done randomly and with intervals of rest—a close simulation of the way our ancestors exercised.

Intrigued, I did some research and learned about the diet and lifestyle components of Evolutionary Fitness and similar plans like the Paleo Diet, the Primal Blueprint, the Caveman Diet, and Ancestral Health.

These plans are all based on the idea that the evolution of human genes has not kept up with the pace of our technology. The advent of agriculture around 10,000 years ago and the subsequent development of mass-produced processed foods introduced humans to a new way of eating that would have been unknown in a natural environment.

Ancestral Health incorporates the added factor of *deep wisdom* with respect to the knowledge that the human inhabitants of a particular environment learned and passed down over great spans of time. We can learn from our ancestors how best to exploit natural plant and animal sources in the pursuit of a more optimal or ideal health—just as we know from them what's poison, and what's food.

I was fascinated by this approach to diet and lifestyle. The basic premise was that to lose weight, people needed to lose the processed foods, reducing the caloric overload (real quality food satiates, and people naturally eat less), and start eating more natural sources of protein and fat—just like our lean, strong, Paleolithic ancestors did.

I dove into it, and my net weight loss rate immediately doubled. Within a few months I discovered **intermittent fasting (IF)** thanks to Art's mention of it, as well as Brad Pilon, author of EatStopEat. I will address the specifics of IF later in the book, but for now, understand that it's simply a recognition that humans are highly adapted to periods of hunger. Without a refrigerator, pantry, and supermarket around the corner, humans were built to go hungry periodically. It's theorized that short periods of hunger can actually be beneficial to our cells. Fasting is, in a word, cleansing.

The fasting helped reprogram my appetite. I began eating a more "carnivorous" diet— reasonably high in fat from mostly animal sources, low to moderate in carbohydrate, and moderate in protein. I included some nuts, but often ate little in the way of fruits or vegetables at first. I had read the plans, but I wasn't following some dietary prescription. I was following my own hungers and desires.

That's right. I let *my own hunger* and my body's signals determine what I ate, and when. I never counted or measured anything. My diet has continued to change over time. There's only one rule: *eat real food*.

In the process of eating real food, I've lost 60 pounds and gained significant strength. I've normalized my blood pressure, I no longer take allergy medication, and I'm off of heartburn medication. I have improved blood lipids, with HDL ("good cholesterol") that runs in the 120s and triglycerides under 50. I have better sleep patterns and better self esteem.

I'm never going back to the SAD. Instead, I'm revealing my secrets so that you, too, can escape from the processed and fast food culture and see the benefits. When the weight starts falling off, you won't need to keep reading mainstream nutrition advice, and you won't need an "expert" to tell you what's healthy. *Your body and your unleashed animal intuition will be the only guide you need*.

9 Points to a Paleo Solution

The Paleo/primal/ancestral lifestyle does not require any counting or macro-nutrient apportioning, and is flexible enough to allow you to eat what you desire amongst a vast array of cooked and raw foods. You'll feast on nutritionally dense animal sources and fiber-rich plant sources.

In fact, Paleo is not really a diet. Rather, it is a *framework* rooted in evolutionary biology within which individuals determine their own lifelong, sustainable regimes.

Here's a 9-point summary of what forms the essence of the approach:

1. **Eat real food.** This includes meat, fish, fowl; natural fats from animals, coconuts, nuts and olives; and veggies and fruits. Add a little dairy if you like it and can tolerate it (butter and cream, especially). Find the balance that works best for you in terms of fat, protein, and carbohydrate ratios. Mix things up seasonally if you can. Consider supplementing with omega-3 fats. Cut out grains, sugar, and vegetable and seed oils. Cut out all processed food in boxes, bags, and cans derived in large measure from these cheap and nutritionally vapid industrial sources.

2. **Avoid drinking calories.** Sodas go without saying, but fruit juice is basically the same, with a little nutrition thrown in. Then there are the various shakes & smoothies. And alcohol. Chewing your nutrition will make a huge difference in your satiation, and it will show up in your body composition.

3. **Allow yourself to go hungry every day, at least a little.** The first meal of the day is a good time—don't eat until you're truly hungry. Every once in awhile, go hungry for a whole day.

4. **Get sensible sunlight exposure.** We evolved outdoors, in the sun. Much like plants need photosynthesis, we need the sun and its vitamin D synthesis on our skin. You should probably get extra vitamin D through supplements. Vitamin D is actually not a vitamin, but a proto-hormone with many functions. It's generally not available in the diet, with the exception of small amounts in things like fish livers.

5. **Run very fast sometimes, play hard when you can, and push and lift heavy**

things around when you have the urge. Do it briefly and intensely; not too often, and not too long. Once to twice per week, for 20–30 minutes each, is plenty. But always push yourself for that brief time. Always try to work out hungry, just like animals hunt hungry.

6. **Allow yourself to be cold sometimes.** Take a cold bath and experience the elements. Or a cold shower. Go out without a jacket.

7. **Go barefoot when you can.** We evolved feet with complex and numerous nerve endings to provide sensory feedback to your brain. You can walk around the house... or be even more adventurous by walking the dogs barefoot, as I do. It connects you to your surroundings.

8. **Get lots of sleep.**

9. **Have sex.** Evolutionarily, it's the only reason we're here, which means it's integral to our very being. Modernity has afforded us means by which sex can be enjoyed privately in many ways, without fear of societal judgment. Whatever it is you like, go for it and enjoy it.

Maybe you're reading this because you're overweight and you're losing hope, or you love a friend or family member who's struggling. You see conflicting information in the media on a daily basis about what is healthy and what is harmful. You've been following your nutritionist's advice and living by the FDA food pyramid like you've always been told to do, but you just keep gaining weight.

I am here to tell you that change is possible. By following the steps laid out in this book, **you will lose fat, gain muscle, and free the animal inside you.**

Become a Hyperink reader. Get a special surprise.

Like the book? Support our author and leave a comment!

III.

Your Inner Animal

Eating Like Our Ancestors

Humans are animals. The same forces of physiology, biology, climatology, geology, and sociology that determine health and prosperity throughout the animal kingdom apply equally to humans.

But unlike non-human animals, humans manipulate nature and their environment. The ability to "create reality" by means of our powerfully creative human minds *is a double-edged sword*.

Man can put reason to work to solve the problem of survival. He can build shelter, fashion clothing, generate heat and other forms of energy, rapidly transport himself over great distances, and even modify the environment to better suit his survival (such as building bridges and dams).

He can also invent or cultivate foods that 3.5 million years of evolution never adapted our genes to handle, or to handle *in concentrations* available today. When you look around and witness the increasing and alarming levels of obesity, diabetes, hypertension, heart disease, and cancer, it becomes increasingly difficult to buy the notion that it's simply a matter of cheap food, sloth, and eating too much.

For the last 30–40 years, since the McGovern Commission and subsequent FDA Guidelines went into effect, people have replaced fat calories with sugar calories (that includes: grain, sugar and vegetable oil-based processed foods in boxes, bags, cans, jars and the freezer section), and the results have been an unmitigated disaster.

What We Can Learn From Animals

Non-human animals in the wild don't become obese or die from unnatural causes without human intervention. Pets and zoo animals under the stewardship of human animals become debilitated when they are fed the wrong foods and subjected to unsuitable environments. Humans become stressed, depressed, unfulfilled, unproductive, dependent, sexually starved, uncompetitive, and unhappy for the same fundamental reasons.

The human animal can live a long and productive life without the decline we now associate with age in modern society. It is possible to experience health, vitality, and happiness right up until the last few days, hours, and even minutes of life. Encoded in our genes is the ability to survive and thrive to the very end on a wide range of food sources.

Good health is natural. It's not something that needs to be industrialized or drug-induced. By eating natural foods available to us, humans can enjoy good health and longevity. Technology should not separate us from or destroy the natural or man-made habitats we and non-human animals need to live and thrive in good health.

The key to being lean, strong, and healthy is in your head. *Use your intuition,* just like animals do. There is no definite prescription or proscription that will work for everyone. You must craft your own diet, health, and fitness paradigm from your own trial and error experience. You must learn to regulate your hunger and satiation. The burden is squarely upon you. Modern institutions only want to sell you stuff. They don't care about your belly or your health. They care about *their* bottom line and *your* spending.

Eating Like Our Ancestors

My diet is omnivorous, and here's why: *human animals are omnivores.* This is a simple fact, accepted by the vast majority of biologists and anthropologists worldwide, and for good reason. Geographic and climatological upheaval over millions of years caused humans to migrate to and inhabit all corners of the globe, from equator to arctic, from seashore to elevations of 16,000 ft. It was essential for humans to evolve the capacity to exploit food sources from a wide range of plants and animals alike. I take full advantage of that.

We can also look to our ancestors to understand how to properly condition our bodies for natural, animal-like physical health. As Chris Shugart at T-Nation writes, quoting Art De Vany, ". . . you should live more like an animal, a human one whose long existence on Earth was spent as a hunter-gatherer. Train, eat, and play, but do it in an intermittent and unpatterned way, just as wild animals do."

There are numerous examples of primitive people who have been studied, who equally enjoy good health. Their diets vary dramatically, but they all include animal products. The archaeological record is clear. We can also learn from examples of modern hunter-gatherers and other non-industrial people.

For a quick example of extremes, let's consider the vastly different diets of the tropical Kitavans and the Arctic Inuit. Kitavans eat about 70% of their energy as carbohydrates, primarily in the form of starchy tubers. The Inuit, on the other hand, have a very low carbohydrate intake, instead getting 70% or more of their energy from animal fat. Both populations typically reach advanced age in excellent health, presenting with none of the diseases of civilization such as diabetes, heart disease, cancer, autoimmune disorders, and others.

Is it true, what Hobbes wrote, that life for the primitive man was "nasty, brutish and short?" Back in the 1920s and 30s, an American dentist, Weston A. Price, concerned with the astronomical rate of tooth decay in his young patients, set out around the world to find out why. Rather than attempt to discover the cause directly, he devised a different approach. What if there were populations of peoples who didn't have tooth decay? If so, then what is it they had that we didn't? His world travels took him to remote places to visit populations of peoples with little to no contact or trade with the modern world, including the Lötschental in Switzerland, Native Americans, Polynesians, Pygmies, and Aborigines, among many others.

What he found was little to no tooth decay in every primitive population studied, at a time when teenagers were being fitted for dentures. His travels are documented in hundreds of photos and pages in his 1939 book, Nutrition and Physical Degeneration. The takeaway message? Modern foodstuffs, concocted largely of various clever proportions of cheap white flour and sugar, were crowding out the dense plant and animal nutrition "primitive" peoples had wisely learned to eat over hundreds or thousands of years of trial and error, in the pursuit of their optimal human animal existence.

For more information concerning the generally good health of "primitive" populations, consult this article by Sally Fallon Morell of The Weston A. Price Foundation (WAPF): Nasty, Brutish and Short? And in regard to the distinction between a wild Paleo existence and that of Ancestral health that seeks to optimize nutrition in a specific environment, see Chris Masterjohn's essay, Understanding Weston Price on Primitive Wisdom.

What's ideal? Who's to say? Your only task is to find what's ideal for *you*, and the options are open-ended.

The Ethics of Eating Animals

For some people, the issues surrounding what to eat go beyond the issue of fat loss or general health. This book makes the case that an appropriate animal based diet is more nutritionally dense, and thus, healthier than any variants of vegetarianism, including the most extreme form: veganism. But there are still those who would avoid animal foods on so-called "ethical" grounds. I don't buy it.

A recent *New York Times* article framed the issue like this:

"In recent years, vegetarians—and to an even greater degree vegans, their hard-core inner circle—have dominated the discussion about the ethics of eating. From the philosopher Peter Singer, whose 1975 volume Animal Liberation *galvanized an international movement, to the novelist Jonathan Safran Foer, who wrote the 2009 best seller* Eating Animals, *those who forswear meat have made the case that what we eat is a crucial ethical decision. To be just, they say, we must put down our cheeseburgers and join their ranks.*

"In response, those who love meat have had surprisingly little to say. They say, of course, that, well, they love meat or that meat is deeply ingrained in our habit or culture or cuisine or that it's nutritious or that it's just part of the natural order. Some of the more conscientious carnivores have devoted themselves to enhancing the lives of livestock, by improving what those animals eat, how they live and how they are killed. But few have tried to answer the fundamental ethical issue: Whether it is right to eat animals in the first place, at least when human survival is not at stake."

The answer to this question isn't difficult. Notions of ethics—the right or wrong of things—must logically begin by asking, What *kind* of animal is the human being? What are we naturally meant to eat?

Again, paleo-anthropology tells us that humans have always eaten meat. From Kleiber's Law—which demonstrates that the chief metabolic difference between humans and our primate ancestors is the tradeoff between brain and gut size—to archaeological digs with piles of scavenged bones, to isotope analysis of fossilized teeth: everything points to an evolution where the hunting and eating of nutritionally dense animals was key in human survival and its ultimate success in becoming a nutritional generalist.

How, then, can vegetarians say that behavior so integral to the success of a species of animal is *wrong*?

Think of it this way: Our sense of right and wrong and our consumption of other animals evolved together, and together made us human. It's all baked into the cake: meat gave us the nutritional density to evolve big brains, big brains gave us the intelligence to introspect, and conscious introspection gave us ethics. *Eating meat made us ethical beings.* Eating meat, therefore, cannot logically be unethical.

The truth is, there's no debunking Paleo. Paleo is more than a mere diet. It's a framework that has supported human life for hundreds of thousands of years—and is thus not a "fad diet" as you'll often see and hear in the media. Our ancestors evolved eating a wide variety of animal and plant matter. That's simply a fact.

Don't let anyone shame you, or make you feel guilty for your own desires and choices. You are a human animal with the freedom to contemplate using the widest array of plant and animal foods you can to find your own sweet spot.

The choice is yours. You can live a life of restriction, denial, hunger, and potentially far more serious long-term problems—or you can discover your own "diet" for life within the framework of a real-food paradigm.

Additional Resources

- Mark Sisson's Primal Blueprint 101

- Arthur De Vany's Evolutionary Fitness Essay

Become a Hyperink reader. Get a special surprise.

Like the book? Support our author and leave a comment!

IV.

The Standard American Diet And Other Diet Health Disasters

Modern Day Diets Are Health Hazards

Here's a look in general terms at just *what we're up against*, folks.

The American Dietetic Association (ADA) supposedly exists to guide the public, by means of its registered dietitians, toward better nutrition—presumably leading to lean, attractive, and healthy bodies.

Under the heading, "Back To Basics For Healthy Weight Loss," the ADA recommends structuring your diet around the following food choices:

- Fruits and vegetables from the produce aisles

- Whole grains from the bakery

- Low-fat milk products from the dairy case

- Lean proteins from the meat/fish/poultry department

If you've ever read mainstream nutrition articles or diet plans, this probably sounds very familiar. And if you've actually tried eating this way, you've probably gotten very frustrated. You've probably realized that eating this way leaves you feeling hungry, physically weak...and most likely, *heavier than ever*. This is especially true when you throw in all the processed "food" that comes in boxes and bags, the sugar-laden drinks, and the fast food that most people consume regularly now.

That's because the people who recommend this approach to food have failed to examine nature and extrapolate a likely diet in light of humans as animals, who evolved over millions of years eating real food—like meat, fish, fowl, natural fats, vegetables, fruits, and nuts. Humans did not evolve over millions of years eating processed grains, vegetable and seed-based *Frankenfats*, meal replacement bars, or low-fat meat and cheese.

In fact, unless one really digs into natural starches from tubers and roots, or pigs out on fruit, it's hard to eat high-carb *and* low-fat on a natural, real foods diet.

Why Could a Processed Food, High Grain and Sugar Diet Be So Dangerous To Health?

Let's look to our ancestors for the answer. According to Mark Sisson of Mark's Daily Apple:

"We humans had the pleasure and occasional scourge of evolving within a hunter gatherer existence. We're talking some 150,000 plus years of hunting and foraging. On the daily scavenge menu: meats, nuts, leafy greens, regional veggies, some tubers and roots, the occasional berries or seasonal fruits and seeds that other animals hadn't decimated. (Ever seen a dog at an apple picking?) We ate what nature (in our respective locales) served up. The more filling, the better."

Going even further back, the primitive ancestors of humans ate this way for at least 2.5 million years. Grains never played any significant role in diet.

The principle reason ancestors didn't take grains into the diet is because it requires too much work for the reward. Think about how much work it would take to locate and pick wild grains, just to get a handful—a few hundred calories at best. Now, compare that with the effort required to take an animal (small or big, even fish and birds) and the thousands of calories you could get from that.

For example, if we had evolved as grain eaters, our lives would resemble that of a gorilla—pretty dismal by our modern standards. They literally have to eat all the time because the nutrient density of the food they eat is so low. Moreover, look at the size of the gut needed to break down and digest all that fibrous plant matter. So why didn't the gorilla evolve out of such an inefficient nutritional paradigm? Simply because it didn't have to. Evolution is driven by the pressure of survival, often brought up by some sort of natural upheaval that presents an "evolve or die out" scenario. So long as there remains suitable environments in which the gorilla can thrive, the gorilla will exist, just as our other primate cousins exist in various similar environments.

The Advent Of Agriculture

Somewhere along the line our ancestors realized that it's better to lay around most of the time, hunt occasionally, bag the meat and fish, and enjoy life. That is, until about 10,000 years ago, when, as Mark continues:

"... the tide turned. Our forefathers and mothers were on the brink of ye olde Agricultural Revolution. And, over time, grains became king. But, as countless archaeological findings suggest, people became smaller and frailer as a result of this new agrarian, grain-fed existence."

Later, of course, people became bigger—but still frail. In the second part of the 20th century, the American diet was increasingly centered around wheat, corn, and other grains. Fast forward to today's situation: according to the Centers for Disease Control and Prevention (CDC), during the past 20 years, there has been a dramatic increase in obesity in the United States, and rates remain high. In 2010, no state had a prevalence of obesity less than 20%. Take a look at this animated graph they have produced.

How did this happen? It was around 1973 when US Senator George McGovern, himself on the low-fat Pritikin Diet, decided to hold Senate hearings on the dietary habits of Americans. The result of those hearings are what eventually ushered in the FDA Dietary Guidelines For All Americans. For a brief history of the spectacle, Tom Naughton, creator and producer of the documentary film *Fat Head* (available on NetFlix and Hulu) has made available these short clips on YouTube: Big Fat Lies and The McGovern Report.

Let's continue along with Mark Sisson's definitive guide to grains:

"Among my many beefs with grain, the first and foremost is the havoc it plays with insulin and other hormonal responses in the body. . . . We developed the insulin response to help store excess nutrients and to take surplus (and potentially toxic) glucose out of the bloodstream. This was an adaptive trait. But it didn't evolve to handle the massive amounts of carbs we throw at it now. And, yes, we're talking mostly about grains. Unless you have a compulsive penchant for turnips, the average American's majority of carb intake comes from grains.

"... And as for the nutritional value of grains? First off, they aren't the complete nutritional sources they're made out to be. Quite the contrary, grains have been associated with minerals deficiencies, perhaps because of high phytate levels. A diet high in grains may also reduce the body's ability to process vitamin D.

"Why not get the same nutrients from sources that don't come back and bite you in the backside? If you have the choice between getting, say, B-vitamins from chicken or some "whole wheat" pasta, I'm going to say go with the chicken every time. Is pasta cheaper? Yes. Is it healthier? No. The B6 in chicken is more bioavailable, for one. The fact is, you pay too high a physiological price for the pasta source. Let's get this point on the dinner table as well: whatever nutrients you can get from whole grains you can get in equal to greater amounts in other food. In terms of nutrient density, grains can't hold a candle to a diverse diet of veggies and meats."

Even when not considering the problems with grains in terms of gluten, and other lectins, be aware that they are not very nutritious.

Listen, everyone, and listen closely: if you eat grains as a significant part of your diet, you are getting CRAP nutrition as compared to a Paleo-like diet. It's simply a fact, the "healthy-whole" fraud notwithstanding. And if that's not enough to convince you, then ask yourself why virtually all grain products have the word "fortified" stamped on the package. Good nutritional sources need never be "fortified."

How about a visual representation? What if we compare the nutrition in bread to some Paleo foods? To do this, I consulted the USDA and it turns out that they recommend that Americans consume 8 ounces of grains per day, with at least half of them coming from whole grains (which are claimed to be more nutritious). So let's go the distance and just compare all 8 ounces as whole grains with other foods. How about beef liver and salmon? I'll use whole wheat bread as a surrogate for all the ways one can get grains (pasta, processed foods, pizza, burger buns, etc.). Eight ounces of whole grains comes out to 600 calories. We'll compare that 600 calories of whole grains with 200 calories of beef liver (4 ounces) and then 400 calories of salmon (8 ounces).

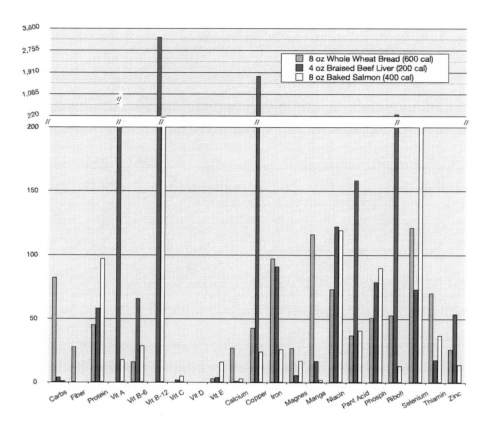

Chart courtesy of Andronique Loannidis, Ph.D., Research Scientist, NanoPower Research Labs. The chart is split due to the "off the scale" nature of some of the nutrient content of beef liver.

As you can see, liver, a mere ⅓ of the energy as the bread—and half that of the salmon —dominates decisively on average (when did you last notice the media or health authorities referring to liver a a "superfood," when, it's the most nutrient dense food on the planet?). The salmon, at ⅔ the energy of bread, dominates the bread. The bread is truly an ugly stepchild.

But let's make it even more dramatic. Since the bread is 600 calories, we can combine the liver and salmon to achieve an equivalent 600 calorie comparison.

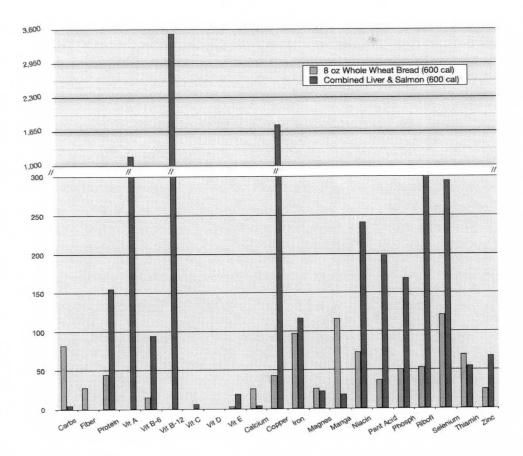

Chart courtesy of Andronique Loannidis, Ph.D., Research Scientist, NanoPower Research Labs. The chart is split due to the "off the scale" nature of some of the nutrient content of the combined liver and salmon.

For a look at the background of the above analysis, see my post at Free the Animal, as well as a more recent, detailed analysis. Let's have some fun with the liver vs. the bread: **2,640% More Nutrition on Average!** No, that's not a typo: Two Thousand, Six-Hundred Forty Percent!, almost 25 times as much nutrition as the bread ounce per ounce. Think of that the next time you hear nonsense about "superfoods"—and it's always some silly berry, or leaf, or something else that while decent, *never* holds a candle to animal foods in terms of nutrition. To repeat, when is the last time you heard of any animal food being referred to as a superfood in any mainstream outlet? Probably never. That's how backwards everything is, and just another example of what you're up against.

Want another example? How about raw oysters on the half shell, which I happen to love. Thing is, it'll be tough for you to get 600 calories worth (remember, the 8 ounces of grains you're admonished to consume). In fact, 24 raw oysters, a large serving indeed, has only 230 calories, about 1/3rd of that 600 calories of whole grains. But guess what? in that 230 calories you'll find 400% of the USRDA for those same 21 nutrients in our comparison. So, one-third the caloric energy, over ten times the nutrition!

But how about if we compare a relatively nutritious plant food to bread? Potatoes are just such a thing. Sweet potatoes are slightly more nutritious than plain white potatoes, so let's use those. Another thing about potatoes in general is that they're gluten free, unlike bread, but—depending on the variety—can have 10—13% protein and it's a quality amino acid profile; whereas, the tiny protein in bread is largely gluten, a big problem for increasing numbers of people. One large sweet potato (excluding any garnishes like butter and not eating the skin) will provide you with 200 calories, one-third of that of our grain recommendation. But the nutrition over those 21 nutrients is 25% of your USRDA. Yes, one potato per day gets you 25% of your nutrition. If you were to eat three of them —in order to match the caloric energy of the bread—you'd get 75% of your USRDA, or roughly twice what you'd get with the grains. ...For centuries, potatoes have been considered a poor man's food, yet their nutritional density is such that eating *only 1/4th of an average male's daily caloric requirement of 2,400 calories* gets you to 75% your recommended allowance in vitamin and mineral nutrition! Bread or grains, on the other hand, are the *true poor man's food.*

Moreover, if your diet is high in grains, the phytic acid you are taking in is causing you to sacrifice your ability to absorb minerals. You are potentially setting yourself up for arterial calcification later in life. This is contributed to by the vitamin D deficiency that goes hand-in-hand with a high grain diet.

The nutritional deficit from grains pushing out far more nutritious and bio-available foods, like meat, fish, veggies, and fruits is the prime reason why they ought to be avoided in any important quantity. If you need more convincing, consider that, as Mark points out:

"Grains, new evolutionarily-speaking, are frankly hard on the digestive system. (You say fiber, I say unnecessary roughage, but that's only the half of it.) Enter gluten and lectins, both initiators of digestive mayhem, you might say. Gluten, the large, water-soluble protein that creates the sludge, err, elasticity in dough, is found in most common grains like wheat, rye and barley (and it's the primary glue in wallpaper paste).

"Researchers now believe that a third of us are likely gluten intolerant/sensitive. That third of us (and I would suspect many more on some level) 'react' to gluten with a perceptible inflammatory response. Over time, those who are gluten intolerant can develop a dismal array of medical conditions: dermatitis, joint pain, reproductive problems, acid reflux and other digestive conditions, autoimmune disorders, and Celiac disease. And that still doesn't mean that the rest of us aren't experiencing some milder negative effect that simply doesn't manifest itself so obviously."

I urge anyone who's interested to read Mark's entire post on grains.

It's Time To Look Out For Your Own Best Interests

Are you convinced yet that grains are basically junk that barely pass for "food?" Yet, this is what the authorities advise that you eat *as your primary source of "nutrition!"* Why?

One reason is that animal products have that "dreaded" fat in them. You've already seen that there's simply no valid comparison in terms of overall micronutrient nutrition, so even if—*if*—there were valid reasons to avoid the devil of saturated fat, one must honesty wonder: *but at what cost?* It doesn't make sense.

Another reason grain is said to be healthier than animal fat—the real reason, in my opinion—is that if you do a little research, you'll find that the ADA is in the pay of the world's leading companies promoting and profiting from obesity and ill-health by producing cheap, highly-processed "food."

You have to dig deep, but if you look at the fine print of any alphabet soup "health" institution website, you can usually find who's paying them to admonish you with unhealthful advice.

- The American Dietetic Association is sponsored by Aramark, Coca-Cola, Hershey, National Dairy Council, Abbott, CoroWise, General Mills, Kellogg's, Mars, Pepsico, Unilever, Soyjoy . . . you get the idea.

- The American Diabetes Association's list of sponsors is essentially the same, with the big drug companies thrown in.

Do you think these companies are paying the ADAs to *diss* sugar-water drinks, processed foods and other sources of poor or bankrupt nutrition, yet high in caloric energy? And if not, how kindly are the ADAs going to take to having its affiliated dietitians and nutritionists contradicting ADA guidelines and policy? How could ADA guidelines and policy possibly be contradictory to the interests of the ones paying the bills?

The ADAs say low fat is good? Then food manufacturers deliver. They line the shelves with products that are low in fat, but high in sugar. The ADAs say whole grains are healthy? Then food manufacturers line the shelves with appealing—to many—products based on grains, and—bonus!—low in fat!

The ADAs say butter is bad? Then food manufacturers give you margarine for decades. But then . . . oops! Margarine contains trans fats, which are now universally recognized as poison. Alright, so they created a whole new line of synthetic "spreads" based on vegetable oils—formerly used as industrial machinery lubricants—extracted by heat and petroleum solvents that have to be deodorized to eat (mouth watering, isn't it?). Hopefully it won't take another four decades to determine that the spreads are as bad, or worse, than the margarine they replaced. *And what will they think of next?*

In light of this, does it not follow that if those same food companies paying the bills have interests that are in conflict with *your* interest in lean, attractive health, that there's actually an antagonism between you and the ADA and their dietitians? Who do you think is going to win out on that one? The whole world of conventional "wisdom" nutrition and dietetics is like the McDonald's chain, because the advice is exactly the same worldwide and for all.

Got that? Does this begin to give you a clue that "experts" and "authorities" might—just maybe—not have your personal best interests at heart as much as their own interests?

What About Vegetarianism and Veganism?

First, it's important to draw a clear distinction between vegetarianism and veganism: vegetarians traditionally consume nutritionally-dense animal nutrition in the form of eggs and dairy. Vegans do not. Nutritionally, this makes a world of difference. Either you consume animal products or you don't, and that's the real distinction to understand.

Some vegetarian societies, such as India, have thrived for millenia, but there has never been any such thing as a vegan society. A fruit-based, raw vegan diet that excludes all animal nutrition is only theoretically possible in narrow, niche environments, such as a rain forest. I say "theoretical," because even supposed primate herbivores are omnivorous. They eat bugs, worms, grubs and termites, and sometimes turn to actual predation and eating of other primates.

You're already familiar with the nutritional comparison of bread versus animal nutrition and even potatoes. But how about fruit? While fruit is indeed a Paleo food, is it suitable as your *only* food? Some people think so. So let's see.

The blog post in question was the result of a live Internet debate I had with a raw fruitarian vegan in April of 2011, with 1,000 people listening in on phone lines and many others streaming live over the internet. During that debate, I issued a challenge to vegans: compare a meal of just fruit to a meal of just beef liver, nutritionally. One vegan took up the challenge and this was the result: Nutrition Density Challenge: Fruit vs. Beef Liver. The comparison took place in two parts. The first part sought to find out how much raw fruit (various, mixed) would be required to roughly equal the vitamin and mineral profile for only 4 ounces of beef liver. The answer is that *it took 5 pounds and 850 calories of fruit to roughly equal the nutrition of 4 ounces and 150 calories of beef liver!*

But who eats only 150 calories for a meal? What happens if, in addition to the liver, we add a sweet potato, some eggs, and fruit—in order to get to an equivalent 850 calorie meal? Then, how about if we construct a varied vegan 850 calorie meal consisting of bread, hummus, almonds, tofu and fruit to achieve a ratio of macronutrients that are about 60% carbohydrate, 20% protein and 20% fat?

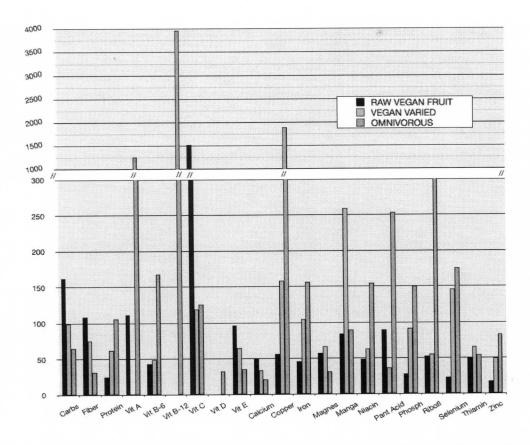

Chart courtesy of Andronique Loannidis, Ph.D., Research Scientist, NanoPower Research Labs. The chart is split due to the "off the scale" nature of some of the nutrient content of the omnivorous meal and in the case of 5 pounds of fruit, vitamin C content.

Here's how these meals stack up:

- 850 Cal Mixed Raw Fruit: 127% USRDA (4 of 21 nutrients over 100%)

- 850 Cal Varied Vegan Meal: 76% USRDA (5 of 21 nutrients over 100%)

- 850 Cal Omivorous Meal: 440% USRDA (12 of 21 nutrients over 100%)

Yes, indeed, in the raw fruit meal there are only 4 of the 21 nutrients that provide 100% or more of the RDA, but 3 of those 4, just barely (vitamin C being the only one that's off the scale). So in essence, a single nutrient at 1,500% of the RDA skews the whole analysis pretty badly. If we were to take vitamin C out of the equation and just average the other 20 nutrients, the fruit meal provides only 57% of the RDA and if you do the same for the varied vegan meal, you still get almost the same average nutrition (74%) so overall, it's really superior to the raw vegan meal overall. However, we do not have nearly this same problem with the omnivorous meal, because 12 of the 21 nutrients are over 100% and of those, 5 are off the scale. Just removing vitamin C as we did in the fruit meal changes nothing at all, because the general nutrition is excellent and widespread. Even if we remove the strongest outlier (B-12), averaging the other 20, we're still at 2.5 times the RDA (263%).

This is a very sad reality for vegans: bankrupt nutrition.

Vegans are experimenting with their lives to a profound degree, far beyond just tweaking a variable or two. Rather than eliminating the most egregious neolithic agents, like wheat, sugar and high-omega-6 industrial oils, they eliminate everything our ancestors ate going back more than 4 million years. The vegan diet requires the massive destruction of habitat for "fields of grain," modern processing techniques, and delivery to markets far far away. Vegans hardly live in the pristine natural paradise they try to sell you on.

Veganism in general, and raw veganism in particular, is a recent human phenomenon that constitutes a mass nutritional experiment with its basis more in ideology, feeling, and myth than in biology, physiology, and nutrition. Vegans begin, as do many Western religions, with their own version of the doctrine of Original Sin.

They try to make you believe that you're guilty by nature. You love the taste and smell of grilling animal flesh, and that makes you a bad person. Vegans sacrifice their desire to eat flesh in favor of "higher ideals"—*as if there was any ideal higher than to live the life of a human animal on Earth as nature has suited.*

Those listening to the "experts" or buying into fundamentalist vegan ideals are getting fatter and sicker. If you forget what you've learned from the ADA and mainstream nutritionists, self-experiment with the lifestyle you were born to live, and follow your instincts to eat real food, the pounds will start melting away and your health will improve immensely.

Additional Resources

- The Bible of the vegetarian and vegan zealots is, of course, *The China Study*, by T. Colin Campbell. For an exhaustive series of critiques of the book using Campbell's methods to statistically analyze the Actual China Study Monograph data, see Raw Food SOS, blogged by statistics geek Denise Minger.

- Want more proof that a diet with any significant grain content is nutritionally inferior, and woefully so? See this post at Free the Animal comparing an average day's nutrition for a SAD eater with that of a Paleo eater.

See also:

- The Vegetarian Myth, by 20-year vegan Lierre Keith

- Vegetarian and Vegan Posts

Become a Hyperink reader. Get a special surprise.

Like the book? Support our author and leave a comment!

V.

Fat Is King

Fat As The 'Good Guy'

People I haven't seen in a while often comment on all the weight I've lost. I love telling them my secret: first and foremost, I eat lots of fat. **Saturated fat,** such as lard, butter, coconut oil, ghee, red palm oil, and olive oil.

Why? As I've discussed, if you want a lean body, you've got to cut the processed foods. Regular and excessive sugar consumption—primarily in the form of drinks with almost no nutritional value—day in, day out drives up baseline insulin to chronically higher levels. It's postulated among many diet doctors and nutritionists that *chronically* elevated insulin levels can drive drive fat storage, as well as inhibit mobilization of stored fat from cells to fuel our activities.

Protein alone doesn't cut it, either. Fat has more than twice as many calories per gram than protein or carbs (nine vs. four). Fat calories are most efficient in terms of volume. Plus, fat makes everything taste better.

For most people, it just doesn't compute. But think about it: fatty meats and eggs are wonderful, nutritious foods with literally millions of years of **evolutionary credentials,** not to mention the *visceral* pleasure almost anyone in their right mind gets from eating them. Yet they get tossed aside by self-important minions.

And who are the self-important minions? *The experts who have been telling us for years that fat is unhealthy, that's who.* The ones who have blood on their hands, as far as I'm concerned. They have, through their arrogant ignorance and disregard for the unassailable logic of human evolution, condemned millions upon millions to moribund lives of physical unattractiveness, obesity, diabetes, heart disease . . . and the list goes on.

As we can see by looking around or looking it up, the statistics get worse year after year, in the very face of the experts' changing advice. But do they ever show humility? No, the best we get is more authoritarian arrogance. *"You eat too much. You don't exercise enough. You haven't been listening to us and you're not properly following our diktats."*

Virtually no one succeeds under the current dietary guidelines, short of becoming the nutritional equivalent of a monk or a nun who practices his or her flagellation three times daily. But as you know, nutritionists have relentlessly pursued an agenda at the urging of huge producers of grain and vegetable oils—those same huge producers who fund many of the "studies" that vilify Real Food and supplant it with *Frankenfood*.

Vegetable oils—of the sort that require solvents to extract—have only been around for maybe 100 years or so. Add to that the astronomical increase in the use of refined sugar and high fructose corn syrup. Throw in the plethora of derivative crap in every packaged product now being consumed by the American public, and increasingly the rest of the world. And while obesity and diabetes skyrocket, even in children, guess what? *You are still being told to cut the fat.*

Saturated Fat Is Good For You!

Can you think of a fundamental reason not to expect that saturated fat is healthy and good?

Stop and think about it. Forget everything you think you know—which, if we're talking *knowledge*, is possibly not much, especially if you're just regurgitating what the "experts" say. Why would saturated fat not be healthful, beneficial? Because it's so tasty, and we naturally want to indulge in pleasures from "the devil's playground?" Does that make any sense?

Could it be, rather, that it's *because* it's so good for us that we have a such a taste for it?

Why wouldn't it be healthful, naturally, when you find it in large percentages in the animal fats associated with all meats? Saturated fat is even in the animal fat associated with human meat, in roughly the same ratio as that found in pigs.

If we were all thinking straight—perhaps like hunter-gatherers responsible on a daily basis to look around, observe, think, integrate, plan, and exercise extreme caution when it comes to feeding ourselves—we might scoff at the notion of animal fat being "bad for us."

Would you expect these super-informed and experienced hunter-gatherers to eschew animal products in favor of leaves and various fibers? You wouldn't, would you? What you would expect is for them to go after the most dense nutrition they could safely source: various animals of all kinds, including their fat, their *saturated* fat.

That's what they've been doing for hundreds of thousands of years, which is very clear from the anthropological record. The skeletal remains of primitive hunter-gatherers are larger in stature, with healthier, straighter teeth and wider dental bridges (no braces!) when compared to those of ancient agricultural populations, or even modern humans.

So, given our millions of years of evolution, one would naturally expect saturated fat to be not only "OK," or, "taken in moderation," *but actually healthful!* Really healthful. One would expect it to be quite an astounding shocker if that wasn't so. In fact, the level of unabashed shock at such speculation *should* have been so profound as to have demanded decades of contradictory-free hypotheses, and gold standard research leading up to infallible proof—*before* even giving it a second thought.

Curse those with the audacity to sweep aside 2.5 million years of evolution to implicate as unhealthy a core building block of our very survival as animals in the wild!

Eat Fat To Lose Weight

Fat is king, folks. In terms of evolutionary logic, it has to be. Pound for pound, fat has more than twice the energy of either proteins or carbohydrates. It was treasured above all other energy sources by our primitive ancestors. Next were the organs, and only then, the muscle meat.

All diets are high-fat diets. Let's say you have 50 pounds of excess fat you'd like to lose in order to get down to around 15% body fat, or thereabouts. Assuming you'll be successful, what does that imply? It means, necessarily, that you're going to metabolize 50 pounds of your own fat in order to accomplish your objective.

Even if you attempt do this by means of a "low-fat" diet, it's still high-fat, as you've got 50 pounds or 175,000 calories worth of fat to burn through. If you do it in six months, that's almost 1,000 calories of fat per day. Presuming a basal metabolism of 2,500 calories, and a dietary intake of 20% fat (a "low-fat diet"), you'd be eating 300 calories of fat and 1,200 calories of protein and carbs combined, for a total consumption of 1,500 calories. The remaining 1,000 would be coming from your own fat, released into your bloodstream and metabolized. Out of the total 2,500 calories, 1,300 of them, or about 50%, are *calories from fat!*

. . . And since your own body fat, like that of a pig, is about 35% saturated, one wonders why people aren't afraid to diet, *for fear of clogging their own arteries while releasing all that saturated fat into their bloodstream!*

You've got to burn through your own fat to lose fat, so it stands to reason that a diet that both satisfies your hunger and keeps insulin levels normal so your fat stores can more easily be released is the best strategy you can implement. You're not hungry—or *as* hungry—because you're getting the energy from your own fat.

Someone on a low-fat, balanced, "everything-in-moderation" diet is usually perpetually hungry. The excessively high intake of carbohydrates in the form of grain and sugar based processed foods means that insulin remains chronically elevated and body fat remains locked in. They're hungrier, lose less weight, often lose lean mass, and ultimately fail to maintain the diet. Yes, on a nutritionally dense diet comprised mostly of animal products you're less hungry because you're getting plenty of quality nutrition and if you're in a fat loss mode you're getting plenty of fat—*your own fat!*

Quit dying on crap, people. Live. Eat in luxury. Dump the notion that the eating of animals is the original sin of nutrition, which only serves to make you feel guilty and defeated each time you give in and so enjoy that grilled rib-eye smothered in rich, sweet, garlicky butter. If you didn't feel guilty for so enjoying what's so natural, you could quickly replace all the crap with actual good food. Once you go through the withdrawals (and you will), you can emerge into a world where food is fun and makes you feel genuinely good. It'll make you look a lot better, too.

Additional Resources

- Dr. Uffe Ravnskov, author of The Cholesterol Myths and Fat and Cholesterol Are Good For You, has a three part series on saturated fat at Spacedoc.com.

- Anthony Colpo, author of The Great Cholesterol Con.

Become a Hyperink reader. Get a special surprise.

Like the book? Support our author and leave a comment!

VI.

Not All Carbohydrates are Created Equal

Fat is King. That does not mean that the Paleo lifestyle is necessarily the same as a low-carb diet.

Often when the Paleo approach is described to people, they will instinctively retort, "sounds like Atkins." Dr. Robert Atkins popularized the low-carb diet back in the 1970s, and it just won't die. There's probably good reason for that. Millions of people—especially diabetics—have benefitted from carbohydrate restriction, lost a lot of weight (fat), and experienced improved health.

Eating Paleo is partly about eliminating grains and sugar, but it's different from a typical low-carb diet. Paleo is about real food: meat, fish, fowl, and vegetables and fruits—the higher the quality, the better. Low-carb snack bars, low-carb breakfast shakes . . . or any of the other plethora of low-carb processed products with incomprehensible ingredients lists are not Paleo.

The truth is, people who lose weight by severely restricting carbohydrate do so because they're eating so much highly satiating, nutritionally dense animal fat and protein and spontaneously eating less—not because they aren't eating carbs. Fat and protein are generally more satiating than carbohydrate, so eating a lot of meat usually means you end up eating fewer calories overall.

Many low-carb diets hold that *all* carbs should be restricted instead of digging deeper to distinguish nutritious carbs from empty ones. What low-carb diets don't take into account is that all carbohydrates are not created equal. Carbohydrates with high nutritional density can also be very satiating, and real foods like sweet potatoes, cassava, and yucca are as Paleo as meat. Also, just as there is an important difference between a grassfed ribeye steak and "Steak-umms," so there is a difference between a baked potato and a half-liter of soda pop.

Despite what Atkins enthusiasts might think, humans and their primate ancestors have always eaten carbohydrate. Take, for example, these lean and healthy populations:

- The Kuna diet was composed of 65% carbs

- The Kitavan diet was composed of about 70-80% carbs (more info on health markers here, here, here, here, and here)

- A highland population in Papua New Guinea in the village of Tukisenta that consumes 94.5% energy as carbohydrate, mostly from sweet potatoes. (lean throughout life, both males and females). See from about 22:00m in this video, obesity researcher Dr. Stephan Guyenet's UCLA Ancestral Health Symposium presentation. (See a recently published book, Sweet Potato Power, by Ashley Tudor for an amazing view into the life of this nutrient dense staple.)

These populations learned over the course of thousands of years to exploit their food resources in the most optimal way, and their bodies evolved to make use of the nutrient-rich carbohydrate that made up such a great percentage of their diets. Restricting carbohydrate intake in societies such as these, particularly those in tropical locations, would have probably resulted in starvation.

When we think "carbohydrate" now, we're usually imagining the processed stuff that comes packaged with a plethora of "confounding variables." Essentially, you can take the same wheat-based carbs, toss in some fat, protein and sugar (then the other 2-3 inches of ingredients on the label), and create a myriad of different enticing products to line shelves or to be served up "fresh" at fast food outlets. The textures and flavors can be as different as is a raw oyster to a too-tough steak, and even the macro-nutrient ratios of carb/protein/fat can differ somewhat . . . but the *micro*nutrient profiles will remain the same: crap. Obviously, restricting these types of carbohydrate is going to be good for your body. But it's important not to blindly dismiss all carbs; they don't belong in the same category as natural, nutrient-rich carbohydrate that enhances a Paleo diet.

Food Satiety

Think about it this way: in nature, there are almost no ways to ingest calories without something backing it up like nutrients, fat, or fiber. For example, you might eat 2-3 oranges if they are really good. But you won't eat a dozen or two dozen of them that's required to make an enormous bottle of *100% Pure Orange Juice*. Why? Because the fiber of the fruit serves to satiate you. You know when you've had enough.

The Journal of the American Medical Association recently published a study titled "A Satiety Index of Common Foods," by Dr. SHA Holt and colleagues, which essentially compared how full different carbohydrates make us feel. As Dr. Stephen Guyenet of Whole Health Source summarized,

"...They fed volunteers a variety of commonly eaten foods, each in a 240 calorie portion, and measured how full each food made them feel, and how much they ate at a subsequent meal. Using the results, they calculated a "satiety index," which represents the fullness per calorie of each food, normalized to white bread (white bread arbitrarily set to SI = 100). So for example, popcorn has a satiety index of 154, meaning it's more

filling than white bread per calorie.

"One of the most interesting aspects of the paper is that the investigators measured a variety of food properties (energy density, fat, starch, sugar, fiber, water content, palatability), and then determined which of them explained the SI values most completely."

Now, before you even look, what food has the *off-the-scale, outlier,* lowest palatability on average vs. the highest satiety?

Potatoes, the "enemy" of the low-carb dieter.

There is an enormous distinction to be made between an average daily consumption of 300-400 grams of carbohydrate consumption from crap in a bag or a drive through, and, say, 200 grams of carbohydrate that comes mostly from potatoes or other starchy real food sources. To put them in the same category is just plain wrong.

Food Reward and Palatability

Let's take this discussion a notch deeper and talk about why so many people choose to eat processed carbs instead of real ones. It's called *food reward and palatability.*

The poor quality processed foods of modern society share these characteristics:

1. It's difficult to stop eating them until there's no more left.

2. You can always find room for more, no matter how much you've already eaten. *There's always room for dessert!*

You aren't nutritionally "rewarding" your body by eating these foods, but your body still treats them as rewards, because they are so highly palatable that they throw off your natural appetite start/stop mechanisms.

To take an example we've all experienced, think of your classic backyard BBQ. Now think of a perfect steak. It can be the best steak you ever had. But no matter how delicious you find it, there always comes a point at which you won't eat another bite. You just can't. It has become unpalatable, and there's no additional "reward" for you in taking another bite. But then, you check out the cakes and cookies on the dessert table, and guess what? *You magically have room for dessert.*

Or think about Lays potato chips, or Pringles. It's difficult to stop eating before the whole bag or can is gone. Not only that, they're not very filling, satiating, even though they're calorically dense. You may even eat more of something else to get your fill, once the bag or can has been dispatched. . . . And have you noticed how you eat Lays or Pringles? You begin with a handful or reasonable snack (and if you stopped there, chalk it up to sensible indulgence now and then). But it almost never stops there, does it? *OK, just one more handful or stack.* And then, after a few of these guilty indulgences in a row separated by mere minutes, you're near the bottom of the bag or can and *oh, well, might as well kill it.* You know what I mean, don't you?

This is what is meant by food reward and palatability. Food engineers and grandmothers have become expert in designing foods we not only can't resist, but don't seem to possess the natural wherewithal to stop after a modest indulgence. We never encountered these sorts of foods in nature. Sweet fruit comes the closest, but fruit is seasonal in all but tropical regions. And even still, most people find it difficult to eat real, whole fruit with abandon.

Convenience is also a huge factor in food reward and palatability. If you bake a dessert from scratch at home, the time and effort it takes to make the food prevents most people from indulging too frequently. Baking homemade apple pies, for example, is a lot of work—it's usually an all-day affair reserved for special holidays or events. But most people don't go to the trouble; it's too easy to stock the freezer with a half dozen frozen pies, just a nuking session away, convenient enough for a weeknight dessert.

The same applies to home cooked dinners. Maybe your favorite meal is fried chicken and mashed potatoes, and you make it at home now and then. No matter how enticingly indulgent a one-off home cooked meal is, gaining fat from chronic overeating is not a one meal affair—you'd have to make it pretty often before it started causing problems. But imagine if, instead of cooking your favorite meal, you could just pull up to a drive-through or call for delivery? This is the situation for many, unfortunately.

Moderate Carb Paleo

Ultimately, calories absolutely count. I can't believe I ever fell for the Low Carb Myth (LCM) that they don't. Don't get me wrong, I don't see anything wrong with being LC if that's what you like and it works for you. A Paleo LC diet is very satiating—since it replaces empty calories with nutrient dense fat and protein. But if you want to, it's perfectly fine to eat potatoes—even white rice (cook it in chicken, beef or vegetable stock to up the nutritional value)—and other natural carbohydrate.

I want things as simple and natural as possible. I don't want to count, and I don't want to do nutrient breakdowns for every meal and I don't want you to think you need to do that either. Rather, I want to eat a varied diet and not worry about eating starch or not eating starch. I want to eat Paleo and within that simple real food limitation, eat what I want, when I want.

Let's consider why low-carb diets work for a lot of people but also, for huge numbers, only for a limited time—at which point they "stall," or often put back on a lot of fat.

As I discussed already, LC diets tend to satiate. Let's look at how this might play out, in Occam's Razor style, i.e., *the less assumptions, the better*.

Let's suppose a 250 pound male body, 5' 10", 50 years old, light to moderate activity level. Daily caloric burn is about 3,500 calories.

He goes low-carb. His target is 160 pounds, 90 pounds away...because that's the last time he remembers where a woman approached *him*. He's been told he doesn't need to count calories or anything—that they don't matter, eat to satiety—under a certain set of *proscriptions* having to do with carbohydrate *per se*.

So it's exactly what he does. After the initial water weight loss and adjustment period, he settles in. Since he doesn't count calories, let me do so, hypothetically. . . .
Wow, amazing. He's not doing anything like 3,500 calories per day. Not even close. Eating *ad libitum*, he's naturally consuming about 2,800 calories for a 700 calorie deficit *per day*, or about a pound lost per 5 days (3,500 calories per pound). He feels awesome, great . . . because even though in big caloric deficit, he's still on a very high fat diet and he's not really hungry too often. He's euphoric on fat, his own fat. The pounds are melting off. He's an LC believer for life. It borders on *Enlightenment*. It's tantamount to a religious experience.

This goes on for just short of a year. He's livin' it up, low-carb style. He's doing himself, friends, and family a huge favor. Don't discount that. But in the end, he's accountable mostly to himself, and in that end, he stalls. He stalls, not at his 160 pound goal where hot chicks might once again approach him, but at 180 pounds, 20 pounds away. He's gonna have to do something, or settle for 2nd string in the chick department.

How can this be? *Low carb is magic.* **He's proved it.** *Over the space of an entire year!*

. . . Or so he thinks.

What he only proved, however, is that *calories count.* Yea, he may have gorged on the fatty meat one night to the tune of pounds and huge calories (and couldn't wait to tell you). But like my dear late grandmother only ever told us about her *jackpots* at the slots —and never the amount she fed it regularly—what he *didn't* tell you is that the next day, he didn't eat much at all. He was satiated. It all subtracts down, over time.

As it turns out, 2,800 average daily calories is about the requirement for a 50 year old guy, 180 pounds, 5' 10", who gets off his ass now and then....Unfortunately, fantasizing about the hot chicks in waiting doesn't burn a whole lot.

Are you beginning to see where I'm going? Low carb was indeed effective. But it was only a means to the end that really worked. Actually, two means: his food palatability/reward was diminished, he spontaneously lowered caloric intake to an *ad libitum* level of a 180 pound man (2,800 calories), and he lost the weight. A year later, right on schedule, he weighs 180.

After months and months or years and years of doing the same thing but expecting a different result, he begins to become disillusioned about low-carb. But the blindspot—because *"calories don't count on low carb"*—is that he never tried 2,600 calories daily on average, the requirement for a 160lb man with his parameters. But, had he done that, he'd have been more hungry and low carb is a lot about not having to feel hungry. It's baked into the low carb cake. So low carb failed him?

That's not fair. Low carb did exactly what it was supposed to do for him—once the science is understood and put into context. Low carb righteously and effectively set off a chain of events that led to him reducing intake in order to lose most of the weight he wanted.

For more on my evolved thoughts on these issues, listen to my podcast with the very popular low-carb advocate, Jimmy Moore.

Become a Hyperink reader. Get a special surprise.

Like the book? Support our author and leave a comment!

VII.

The Cholesterol Con

Challenging Mainstream Assumptions

While there's no magic to low-carb/high-fat, it can be very effective for many. Even people who see the excellent weight loss results achieved with such a lifestyle are hesitant to put it into practice. Why?

- They believe that saturated fat causes high cholesterol

- Thanks to decades of being subjected to "expert" opinions, they believe that high cholesterol causes heart disease

By now you know that this e-book is all about challenging mainstream assumptions. With that in mind, take a look at this post and chart on heart disease death stats by country. Which countries do you think have the highest intake of saturated fat?

Showing latest available data.

Rank	Countries	Amount (top to bottom)	
#1	Slovakia:	216 per 100,000 people	
#2	Hungary:	192.1 per 100,000 people	
#3	Ireland:	152.6 per 100,000 people	
#4	Czech Republic:	148.6 per 100,000 people	
#5	Finland:	143.8 per 100,000 people	
#6	New Zealand:	127.3 per 100,000 people	
#7	United Kingdom:	122 per 100,000 people	
#8	Iceland:	115.4 per 100,000 people	
#9	Norway:	112.5 per 100,000 people	
#10	Australia:	110.9 per 100,000 people	
#11	Sweden:	110.1 per 100,000 people	
#12	Austria:	109.3 per 100,000 people	
#13	United States:	106.5 per 100,000 people	
#14	Germany:	106.1 per 100,000 people	
#15	Denmark:	105.4 per 100,000 people	

[Source]

If the "diet-heart hypothesis" were true in its general position on fats, and on saturated fats in particular, then ought we not see some significant correlation between saturated fat intake and coronary heart disease deaths?

In the United States, the average saturated fat intake is estimated at around 12% of total energy. As you can see, we're number 13 on the chart.

Let's talk about a country where it's documented that the population derives 40–50% of its energy, not from just fat, *but from saturated fat.*

Dr. Stephan Guyenet of the blog *Whole Health Source* reports on the dietary habits of the Tokelau Island Migrants, saying that "...[t]hey derive between 54 and 62 percent of their calories from coconut, which is 87% saturated. This gives them perhaps the highest documented saturated fat intake in the world."

"The Tokelau Island Migrant study isn't a perfect experiment, but it's about as close as we're going to get. Tokelauans traditionally obtained 40–50% of their calories from saturated fat, in the form of coconut meat. That's more than any other group I'm aware of, even topping the roughly 33% that the Masai get from their extremely fatty Zebu milk.

"So are the Tokelauans dropping like flies of cardiovascular disease? I think most of the readers of this blog already know the answer to that question. I don't have access to the best data of all: actual heart attack incidence data. But we do have some telltale markers. In 1971–1982, researchers collected data from Tokelau and Tokelauan migrants to New Zealand on cholesterol levels, blood pressure and electrocardiogram (ECG) readings."

The punch line is that the *Tokelauans had ECG readings with 0.0% of men showing markers for a past heart attack,* while substantial numbers of men in New Zealand— where saturated fat intake is 50% less—showed up with the markers. Needless to say, Tokelauans didn't show up on the chart above. Every single hunter-gatherer and other non-industrial population that has been studied directly contradicts the hypothesis that "saturated fat causes heart disease."

In fact, no such causal link has ever been even close to being proved. Even the associations once thought to be solid aren't there.

Stephan does his typical marvelous job in sorting through all the relevant material, so why not go over and have a look at his articles:

- The Tokelau Island Migrant Study: Background and Overview

- The Tokelau Island Migrant Study: Dental Health

- The Tokelau Island Migrant Study: Cholesterol and Cardiovascular Health

- The Tokelau Island Migrant Study: Weight Gain

- The Tokelau Island Migrant Study: Diabetes

- The Tokelau Island Migrant Study: Asthma

- The Tokelau Island Migrant Study: Gout

- The Tokelau Island Migrant Study: The Final Word

Myths About Cholesterol

The same is true of cholesterol. In the United States, where nutritionists dispense reams of dietary advice geared toward lowering cholesterol, and the list of medications intended to "fight" cholesterol just keeps getting longer, *about half the people who die of heart disease have low cholesterol, half high.* For women, higher cholesterol seems to be associated with higher longevity. For older people, too.

Here's a short, 70-second video on YouTube by a medical doctor in the United Kingdom, Dr. Malcolm Kendrick. He simply plotted readily available epidemiological data from the World Health Organization (WHO). The data plots incidence of death from heart disease against average cholesterol levels in the same populations. Do watch the shot video linked above, but here's the punchline in this figure, beow.

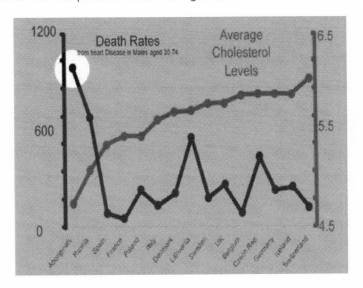

Dr. Malcolm Kendrick Video

Australian aboriginals have the lowest recorded average cholesterol in the world, combined with the highest incidence of death from heart disease. Conversely, the Swiss have the highest recorded average cholesterol in the world, combined with the lowest incidence of death from heart disease.

Case closed. End of story. There's nothing to see here. That's called falsification of a hypothesis.

There's no meaningful association between low-density lipoprotein (LDL) cholesterol (the "bad" cholesterol) levels and heart disease. Time and time again, if hundreds of thousands of heart attack patients are analyzed, half have low LDL and half have high LDL. It's irrelevant.

The LDL cholesterol results you get in your routine blood workup are completely useless. *The important information is not your LDL, but your triglycerides.*

So what are **triglycerides**? Most simply, fat circulating in your blood. Government recommendations are for a level of 150 and below. Mine are habitually around 50, and high-fat (and consequently, low-carb) dieters all have pretty low triglycerides (in the 50–80 area). Eat substantial natural fat (from animals, coconut, and olives) and you'll dramatically reduce your triglycerides, because you won't be hungry for the things that raise them on a daily, 24/7 basis.

Let's back up a second. And unless you're a lab technician, this will likely be news to you: your LDL level—unless you get a direct measurement, which is an expensive test not normally ordered—*is calculated* using the Friedewald equation:

LDL = Total Cholesterol – HDL – (Triglycerides/5)

All else remaining equal, each 5-point increase in Trigs gets you a point off your LDL, whether your LDL really decreases for real or not. Increase Trigs by 100, and you can lower your LDL by 20.

Let's take an example. Suppose your labs come back and you have a rather average lipid panel. That could be a total cholesterol of 225, with its components of HDL, triglycerides and LDL at 40, 225, and 140, respectively. But guess what: only total HDL and trigs were actually measured.

140 = 225 – 40 – (225/5)

Recall that in algebraic notation, the 225 is divided by 5, and the result of that calculation is then subtracted from the total and HDL. All else being equal in the equation, raising that number that's currently 225 will lower the number on the other side, your LDL.

The association between high triglycerides and heart disease is very well established. Even the National Lipid Association, from which this study and statement originate, acknowledges an independent association with triglycerides:

"…triglycerides are the third component of the lipid profile and are an independent and

compounding risk factor for heart disease, the leading cause of death in the U.S. Studies have shown that the risk of developing heart disease doubles when triglyceride levels are above 200 mg/dL. When triglycerides are above 200 mg/dL and HDL cholesterol is below 40 mg/dL, a person is at four times the risk of developing heart disease."

(Curiously, that study or article appears to be no longer available on their website, but thanks the the ever present Google, a report on it was found at Life Extension Europe. I also reported on it at Free the Animal.)

A very high-carb, low-fat diet—the kind prescribed by doctors to lower your LDL—will cause your triglycerides to rise. People who eat lots of grains and sugars in the form of bread, pasta, rice, processed foods, sweetened sodas, and fruit juices have triglycerides levels of 200 and on up; 300–400 and above are not uncommon.

So, your doctor (and nutritionist, and every mainstream health writer) tell you to lower your LDL? A six-pack of Coca Cola per day ought to do the trick. Your trigs will skyrocket and your LDLs will absolutely go down, but only because of math, not biology. Your doctor will tell you you're doing a great job, and you can live in ignorant bliss.

Now, with the Friedewald equation in mind, and the foregoing analysis and examples, let's revisit the study from the National Lipid Association via Life Extension Europe:

"A new 30-year analysis of the National Health and Nutrition Examination Survey (NHANES) database conducted by the National Lipid Association (NLA) indicates that while Americans are doing a better job of managing LDL or "bad" cholesterol, the percentage of adults with high triglycerides, a blood fat linked to heart disease, has doubled, leaving many people at risk for potentially life-threatening events such as heart attack or stroke. Results of the analysis were presented today at the American Heart Association's Annual Scientific Sessions in New Orleans."

Now, watch how they can't see the forest through the trees:

"Between 1976 and 2006 the number of Americans with unhealthy isolated LDL levels dropped from 43 percent to 40 percent, an improvement that researchers attribute to more aggressive educational initiatives and treatment. However, far less emphasis has been placed on controlling triglycerides. The rising rates of isolated high triglycerides seen over the last three decades underscore the need for physicians and patients to understand and treat all three key lipids, which include LDL, HDL or 'good' cholesterol and triglycerides."

Get it? They attribute lower LDLs with better education and treatment, when the Occam's razor explanation is that by virtue of the equation they use, *the pure math they use*, the majority of the lowering of LDL is a simple sixth-grade-level calculation having to do with elevated triglycerides. In other words, their "educational initiatives" have been to prescribe low-fat, high-sugar (carbohydrate) diets, resulting in grossly elevated triglycerides, and mathematically lowered LDLs.

This is the outright FRAUD that's being perpetrated against you by "authorities" and "experts"—many in the pay of the drug companies who want you popping statins, that most profitable class of drugs in history, (commonly known as "cholesterol lowering medication"). Do the words Crestor, Lipitor, and Lovastatin ring a bell? You watch TV, don't you?

Listen To Your Body, Not The Numbers

The Paleo diet operates from a principle that has an important basis in fact: we know that we evolved to eat plants and animals. We know the archaeological record shows excellent health enjoyed by pre-agricultural humans, provided their environment was sufficient to meet their needs. We know that dozens, even hundreds of societies of primitive hunter-gatherers, pastoralists, and other non-industrial peoples have been observed by physicians and other scientists going back 200 years, and virtually none of the diseases of civilization show up.

How do you feel? That's the important question. Don't worry about your LDL, because cholesterol is not a problem to be managed. A diet of real foods is what is to be managed, and the cholesterol numbers are just numbers.

Additional Resources

- Dr. Uffe Ravnskov, author of Fat and Cholesterol Are Good For You

- Anthony Colpo, author of The Great Cholesterol Con

- Dr. Malcolm Kendrick, author of The Great Cholesterol Con (same name, different book)

- Dr. Malcolm Kendrick and Dr. Duane Graveline, authors, The Statin Damage Crisis

Become a Hyperink reader. Get a special surprise.

Like the book? Support our author and leave a comment!

VIII.

Natural Disease Prevention

Paleo Power: Preventing Allergies, Diabetes, & Cancer

I've been a seasonal allergy sufferer all my life, since my teenage years. This used to be debilitating in the spring and summer. Eventually, I found it was just best to take the prescriptions year round, it was so bad. Same with acid reflux: I get nuclear heartburn. In the past, I was forced to fall back on medications to ease the symptoms.

Since I went grain-free and Paleo in general, I have stopped taking allergy medication. I've just sailed through spring and summer, never once feeling the urge to renew my old prescriptions. I still get mild heartburn from time to time, but it's always directly related to consuming food or drink outside of the Paleo lifestyle.

I've discussed the ways in which the Paleo lifestyle prevents obesity, diabetes, hypertension, heart disease, stroke and other problems that are commonly known and referred to as *Diseases of Civilization.* But there are even more health benefits you'll enjoy if you start eating a Paleo diet.

To begin with, you'll experience increased energy levels and better health in general, on a daily basis. You'll sleep better and be less prone to minor headaches and stomach upsets. You'll have sex as gobsmacked exciting as you had as a teenager or young 20-something.

Research shows that the Paleo lifestyle can also be an effective strategy against debilitating conditions like diabetes and even cancer. You might be skeptical of this claim at first, but think about it: diabetes and cancer are modern diseases that our Paleolithic ancestors rarely experienced. It makes sense that returning to their natural, instinctive way of eating and living could be the right way to prevent and cure conditions caused by unnatural exposures and behaviors.

Remediation For Diabetes?

It's well known that a diet high in carbohydrates is dangerous for people with type 2 diabetes. The problem is that many doctors also believe that a diabetic meal plan should also be low in fat.

My mom, in her early 70s, is a Type 2 diabetic. I have witnessed that the "help" she used to get from the medical establishment went beyond malpractice. When she was diagnosed some years ago, there was considerable confusion about what she ought to eat. She was aware of the low-carb advice, but her doctors were telling her to eat low-fat —advice that is pervasive throughout the medical community.

As we all know, it is very hard to maintain a low-carb diet that's also low in fat. You have to eat *something*. Making up the difference with protein can get very unpleasant. Just in terms of sheer mass, fat is more than twice as energy efficient as either protein or carbs.

On this recommended low-fat diet, my mom's blood glucose levels kept creeping up. She'd have huge swings, with spikes well over 200 and more. To put that in perspective, a normal pancreas will release enough insulin to keep blood glucose no higher than about 145 mg/dL as an absolute spike; normal is in a range of about 80–100.

Finally, the doctors determined she had to go on the self-administered insulin shots. She's no dummy. She could see the downward progression. Type 2s always get worse and worse.

Then my mom went on a high-fat, super low-carb diet, with no concern for how much fat or she ate. She consumed no grains, no grain products, and very limited fruit. Her blood glucose quickly stabilized between 85 and about 105 most of the time. She had been used to shooting two types of insulin, a fast-acting and a time-release; a few weeks into the new diet, she was able to drop the fast acting one.

Since then, she has been able to reduce the shots to zero (though she keeps the medication handy and current, just in case) and has even been able to reduce the oral medication.

The low-carb, high fat approach is also effective for people with type 1 diabetes. Dr. Richard Bernstein, author of Diabetes Solution, has been living with it for 60 years. As a young man, he was literally dying from the disease and its side effects. Determined that he had to take matters into his own hands, he figured out the diet that would tightly control his incurable condition, and he sought to share it with others. But he was only an engineer, so his admonitions fell on deaf ears. He went back to school and got his MD so someone would listen to him. His website is chock full of both Types 1 and 2s who have helped themselves through exercise and very low-carb dieting to keep their diabetes in check.

Sugar Feeds Cancer

While cancer does exist in the wild, it's an aberration. It's rare. There is also evidence that ingesting sugar (including too much grain, fruit, and juice) in the presence of cancer increases the rate of tumor growth.

Patrick Quillin, PHD, RD, CNS, writes,

"A mouse model of human breast cancer demonstrated that tumors are sensitive to blood-glucose levels. Sixty-eight mice were injected with an aggressive strain of breast cancer, then fed diets to induce either high blood-sugar (hyperglycemia), normoglycemia or low blood-sugar (hypoglycemia). There was a dose-dependent response in which the lower the blood glucose, the greater the survival rate. After 70 days, 8 of 24 hyperglycemic mice survived compared to 16 of 24 normoglycemic and 19 of 20 hypoglycemic. This suggests that regulating sugar intake is key to slowing breast tumor growth.

"In a human study, 10 healthy people were assessed for fasting blood-glucose levels and the phagocytic index of neutrophils, which measures immune-cell ability to envelop and destroy invaders such as cancer. Eating 100 g carbohydrates from glucose, sucrose, honey and orange juice all significantly decreased the capacity of neutrophils to engulf bacteria. Starch did not have this effect.

"A four-year study at the National Institute of Public Health and Environmental Protection in the Netherlands compared 111 biliary tract cancer patients with 480 controls. Cancer risk associated with the intake of sugars, independent of other energy sources, more than doubled for the cancer patients. Furthermore, an epidemiological study in 21 modern countries that keep track of morbidity and mortality (Europe, North America, Japan and others) revealed that sugar intake is a strong risk factor that contributes to higher breast cancer rates, particularly in older women."

Add to this the fact that cancer has been virtually unknown amongst traditional hunter-gatherers and non-industrial peoples. And as we know, sugar was rare in the Paleo. Processed and concentrated sugar products were nonexistent.

If sugar (by which I mean all grains, sodas, juices, and so on) feeds cancer, what happens when cancer patients eliminate it from their diet?

According to Dr. Michael Eades of ProteinPower.com,

". . . Since the cancers can use only glucose, and since glucose is made in the cancer cells slowly and inefficiently, the cancer cells have to rely on outside glucose to provide nourishment for their rapid growth and replication. People on very-low-carb diets produce ketones, which take the place of glucose in other cells that can use these ketones for fuel. But cancer cells can't use the ketones since ketones have to be burned in the mitochondria, which are dysfunctional in cancer cells. If you can keep blood sugar low, then growth of the cancer cells may be held in check long enough for the body's own previously overwhelmed immune system to rally and beat the vulnerable cancer back."

In other words, it may be possible to cure, or at least slow, your cancer by eating a low-carb, high-fat diet.

If indeed this evolutionary, ancestral, primal way of eating—going hungry sometimes and engaging in activity— represents an effective firewall against cancer, then what do you suppose that says about the validity of an evolutionary approach to your life and diet?

Just imagine it. You take a diet that approximates that of pre-agricultural man, i.e., the diet he ate for 2.5 million years—versus the last ten thousand years—and you use it to slow, beat, or prevent cancer.

No miracles or silver bullets. Just a simple and nutritious existence.

Additional Resources

- My Posts on Cancer at Free the Animal

- Does Sugar Feed Cancer?

- Will The Blogosphere Cure Cancer?

- More on Sugar and Cancer

- More on Cancer

- Sugar Feeds Cancer

Going Paleo can Improve Symptoms of Multiple Sclerosis

Let me tell you the story of a medical doctor with advanced multiple sclerosis (MS) who found that living a Paleo lifestyle greatly ameliorated the symptoms of her disease.

According to Wikipedia, "**There is no known cure for multiple sclerosis**. Treatments attempt to return function after an attack, prevent new attacks, and prevent disability. MS medications can have adverse effects or be poorly tolerated, and **many patients pursue alternative treatments, despite the lack of supporting scientific study**" [Perhaps because all "scientific study" is focussed on making big bucks by patenting a pill, and not alternatives to pills [emphasis added].

While I'm not qualified to judge if what Dr. Wahls did for herself constitutes a "cure," she no longer has apparent symptoms, and she did it by dumping the best "care" and drugs available in the world.

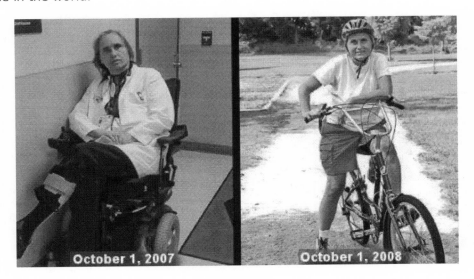

Dr. Wahls

Dr. Wahls tried all the best medications and diets, but she got progressively worse. She decided to stop listening to the advice of "food" manufacturers and the pill pushers, went on a Paleo diet, and got better. Simple as that.

She conducted a clinical trial on herself. Take a look at these shocking results:

"At 3 months, outcome measures improved from baseline as follows: Fatigue Severity Scale by 34.2%, Timed 25 foot walk by 16.6%, Get up and go test by 20.7%, average speed during 25 foot walk test by 20.35% and total Multiple Sclerosis Spasticity Scale (MSSS-88) by 16.3%. At 6 month average improvement of first 3 subjects were as follows: Fatigue Severity Scale by 31.4%, Timed 25 foot walk by 14.4%, Get up and go test by 27.1%, average speed during 25 foot walk test by 17.5% and total MSSS-88 by 26.5%. No significant adverse events were reported. In conclusion, individuals with SPMS are willing to complete a complex behavioral change involving intensive directed nutrition, neuromuscular electrical stimulation and progressive exercise program. Preliminary results indicate beneficial effects of this combined intervention on fatigue and gait in subjects with a progressive disease who are not expected to show improvement."

Dr. Wahls spoke about her experiences at a TEDx presentation in Iowa City in early November.

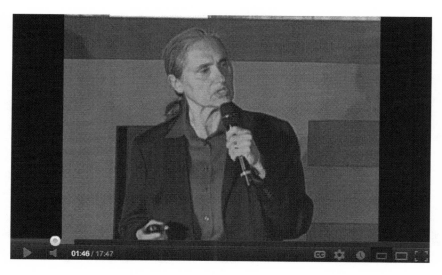

TED talk Iowa City via Youtube

The video is only 17 minutes long, and I encourage you to watch the whole thing. It's really a great encapsulation of what the whole Paleo diet is about from a health and disease standpoint, rather than a weight and fat loss basis. One very telling thing she shows is how most Americans are deficient in an array of essential nutrients and how a proper Paleo diet not only restores adequate nutrition, but delivers up to 10 times the nutrition of the Standard American Diet ("SAD"). It also provides substantially more nutrition than the American Heart Association Diet, American Diabetes Association Diet, the FDA Food Pyramid or anything else you can name. See the chapter on "**The Standard American Diet And Other Diet Health Disasters**" again, if you haven't grasped that, yet.

It's also worth noting from her presentation that gluten proteins in grains and casein in dairy are associated with a wide array of ailments, including but not limited to: eczema, asthma, allergies, infertility, irritable bowel, fibromyalgia, chronic fatigue, arthritis, chronic headache, neurological problems and behavior problems. And yet, how often do you hear much about dietary intervention, as opposed to some new drug therapy? Well, you now have "gluten free," along with the same cast of characters producing essentially the same vapid crap: no gluten, and probably twice the sugar.

Additional Resources:

- Dr. Wahls' website

- Dr. Wahls' book: Minding My Mitochondria: How I overcame secondary progressive multiple sclerosis (MS) and got out of my wheelchair

- More self-reported success stories

The Role Of Vitamin D: Are You A Fish Out Of Water?

Vitamin D deficiency is potentially implicated in just about every modern disease you can name. The problem is due in part to mass modern migration. Dark skin is resistant to ultraviolet sunlight, and thus synthesizes less vitamin D per unit of time than white skin. The lighter the skin, the more efficient the absorption. With people's migration to different regions, dark-skinned people now live at higher latitudes in the northern and southern hemispheres, and lighter-skinned people live at lower ones. This sets up the former for deficiency and the latter for overexposure.

But it seems to me that the former situation is the far riskier one. People with lighter skin can always avoid overexposure, use some sunscreen, etc., but people with darker skin at higher latitudes, such as northern Europe, Northern areas of the US, and Canada, suffer a double whammy of having less efficient skin for synthesis, combined with a sun that's only effective in stimulating vitamin D for part of the year (the higher the latitude, the less effective).

Let's take a look at some research. Previously, there was only a 1971 study conducted on 8 sunbathing, white lifeguards who maintained levels in the range of 50-80 ng/ml, but now there's a good amount of epidemiology for vitamin D levels in people with various illness and disease, and for disease incidence by latitude.

A new study measured the vitamin D levels of the Masai and Hadzabe of Africa. Dr. John Cannell explains the study thusly:

"The Maasai are no longer hunter-gatherers but live, along with their cattle, either a settled or a semi-nomadic lifestyle. They wear sparse clothes, which mainly cover their upper legs and upper body, and attempt to avoid the sun during the hottest part of the day. They eat mainly milk and meat from their cattle, although recently they began to add corn porridge to their diet. Their mean 25(OH) vitamin D level was 48 ng/ml (119 nmol/L) and ranged from 23 to 67 ng/ml."

The health of the Masai, in general, is excellent. Check out Dr. Stephan Guyenet's series to see for yourself:

1. Diet and Body Composition of the Masai

2. Masai and Atherosclerosis

3. More Masai

4. Nutrition and Infectious Disease

That 4th link wasn't actually in the series but deals with the Masai, as well as vitamins A & D, which we now know work in synergy (along with K2). Here's an excerpt:

"…However, their colleagues had previously noted marked differences in the infection rate of largely vegetarian African tribes versus their carnivorous counterparts. The following quote from Nutrition and Disease refers to two tribes which, by coincidence, Dr. Weston Price also described in Nutrition and Physical Degeneration:

"'The high incidence of bronchitis, pneumonia, tropical ulcers and phthisis among the Kikuyu tribe who live on a diet mainly of cereals as compared with the low incidence of these diseases among their neighbours the Masai who live on meat, milk and raw blood (Orr and Gilks), probably has a similar or related nutritional explanation. The differences in distribution of infective disease found by these workers in the two tribes are most impressive. Thus in the cereal-eating tribe, bronchitis and pneumonia accounted for 31 per cent of all cases of sickness, tropical ulcers for 33 per cent, and phthisis for 6 per cent. The corresponding figures for the meat, milk and raw blood tribe were 4 per cent, 3 per cent and 1 per cent.'

"So they set out to test the theory under controlled conditions. Their first target: puerperal sepsis. This is an infection of the uterus that occurs after childbirth. They divided 550 women into two groups: one received vitamins A and D during the last month of pregnancy, and the other received nothing. Neither group was given instructions to change diet, and neither group was given vitamins during their hospital stay. The result, quoted from Nutrition and Disease:

"'The morbidity rate in the puerperium using the [British Medical Association] standard was 1.1 per cent in the vitamin group and 4.7 in the control group, a difference of 3.6 per cent which is twice the standard error (1.4), and therefore statistically significant.'

"This experiment didn't differentiate between the effects of vitamin A and D, but it did establish that fat-soluble vitamins are important for resistance to bacterial infection."

So, there appears to be a dietary factor as well, which should make perfect sense, since we evolved over millions of years outdoors, at latitudes appropriate to our skin's ability to produce vitamin D, and we ate real foods—not nutritionally bankrupt serial grains and all the processed crap they make from them now.

Just one more thing. How about cancer? While I looked but could find no references for cancer rates in the Masai, I do have some epidemiology for various cancers by vitamin D levels as well as latitude.

It's from this very long and complex presentation: Dose-Response of Vitamin D and a Mechanism for Prevention of Cancer (PDF).

This first slide is a plot of renal cancer rates in males (left) and females (right).

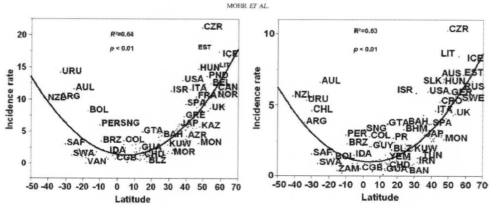

FIGURE 1 – Renal cancer incidence rates, males, by latitude, 2002. Source: Data from GLOBOCAN[1].

FIGURE 2 – Renal cancer incidence rates, females, by latitude, 2002. Source: Data from GLOBOCAN[1].

What do you make of that? Can anyone think of anything that might explain it *better, with fewer assumptions* (Occam's Razor style) than vitamin D?

Dose-response relationships from cohort studies were used to estimate the number and percent of cancer cases that could be prevented worldwide by vitamin D3 supplementation:

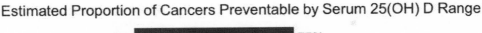

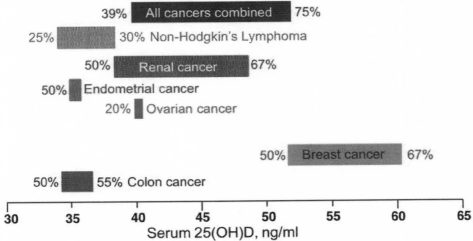

Estimated Proportion of Cancers Preventable by Serum 25(OH) D Range

Basically, what this estimates is that keeping your level of 25(OH) vitamin D level above 50 ng/ml dramatically reduces your risk of cancer.

Given the above, I see no reason anyone should not be setting about to ensure it. *Eat real food while you're at it and better your chances even more.*

Here's the list of cohort studies that were used in that last graph:

- Gorham ED, et al. Am J Prev Med. 2007;32:210-6.

- Garland CF, et al. Am Assoc Ca Res Mtg San Diego April 14, 2008

- Li H, et al. PLoS Med. 2007;4:103.

- Tworoger SS, et al. Cancer Epidemiol Biomarkers Prev. 2007;16:783-8.

- Mohr SB, et al. Prev Med. 2007;45:323-4.

- Mohr SB, et al. Int J Cancer. 2006;119:2705-9.

- Purdue MP, et al. Cancer Causes Control. 2007;18:989-99.

- Lappe JM, et al. Am J Clin Nutr. 2007;85:1586-91.

In sum, I would recommend looking into vitamin D supplementation. We don't live and work outdoors as we evolved to do. Rather, we live in homes, work in offices, and go back and forth in cars, trains, and buses.

The bottom line: it's important to make sure you're getting enough vitamin D, and it's tricky to get it all from the sun. See the chapter on "**Cold Therapy**" for information on vitamin D supplements.

Additional Resources

- My posts on Vitamin D at Free the Animal

- Epidemic Influenza and Vitamin D

- Vitamin D Deficiency and Type 1 Diabetes

- Melanoma, Sun, and Its Synthetic Defeat (Sunscreen)

- Vitamin D Deficiency and All Cancer

- New Research Shows Vitamin D Reduces Risk of Cancer

- The Vitamin D Council

- GrassrootsHealth

Activator X, AKA: Vitamin K2, Menatetrenone

As I mentioned in the chapter on **"Your Inner Animal,"** 20th century dentist Weston A. Price found that 1 in 3 of his patients exhibited crowded, rotten teeth. He traveled the world to find out if there were populations without either of those problems. He found indigenous peoples in generally pristine health. He also tracked down members of these populations who'd left to enter the modern world, finding they'd fallen to the same degraded health and tooth decay that had set him on his journey in the first place.

Price found what I consider to be three very important things: almost no dental cavities (about 1 tooth in 1,000 vs. 1 in 3 in the modern world), wide dental bridges (no need for "braces"), and near effortless childbirth (wide birth canals in females).

There were other differences between indigenous societies and modernized ones. Price found that indigenous peoples enjoyed generally high nutritional density and profound ancestral wisdom. And their methods for acquiring food were quite unlike the robotic routines many of us employ today: drive a cart down the supermarket lane and fill a cart with boxes, bags, cans, bottles, and the ever-present sweet, sugary drinks.

Eat, drink, and repeat.

So what was the magic of indigenous nutrition? It wasn't magic, but logic. If you're not driving a car, parking, driving a shopping cart, using your ATM card and driving back home, you might have to scrounge through the bush, track down prey, kill it, dress it, haul it back to camp, and present it to voraciously hungry souls.

If that's your situation, are you going to toss the liver? Kidneys? How about the heart?

How about the bone marrow? The brain?

Or what about other nutritionally dense offal, such as sweetbreads and the like?

When luxury abounds, waste abounds, and hunter-gatherers didn't have the luxury to waste anything. And it just so happens that the "nasty bits" are the most nutritionally dense, as has been illustrated with liver compared to bread and vegan diets in the chapter on **"The Standard American Diet And Other Diet Health Disasters."**

It turns out that there's a nutrient in such things as liver, fish eggs, and all sorts of things people don't commonly eat anymore, but ate preferentially throughout human evolution.

That nutrient may be what has now been identified as **Vitamin K2,** of which there are many sub-forms. Some K2 sub-forms are found in the tissues of various animals, and others are produced by bacterial fermentation in such things as certain cheeses and natto, a Japanese dish of fermented soybeans.

The jury is still out on which is optimal or whether there's a marked difference, but the history of evolution makes me suspect that the animal forms are what we evolved to eat. Humans are very poor at converting the plant form of vitamin K (K1) to the more active form (K2). But ruminant animals convert it very efficiently, so they eat the greens, produce K2, and we eat them.

Vitamin K2 has been used in relatively high doses to reverse arterial calcification in rodents. And as shown in an excerpt in this post at Free the Animal, Weston Price used a combination of cod liver oil and a special formulation of pastured butter oil to not only halt dental decay, but reverse it:

"Weston Price was primarily interested in Activator X because of its ability to control dental caries. By studying the remains of human skeletons from past eras, he estimated that there had been more dental caries in the preceding hundred years than there had been in any previous thousand-year period and suggested that Activator X was a key substance that people of the past obtained but that modern nutrition did not adequately provide. Price used the combination of high-vitamin cod liver oil and high-Activator X butter oil as the cornerstone of his protocol for reversing dental caries. This protocol not only stopped the progression of tooth decay, but completely reversed it without the need for oral surgery by causing the dentin to grow and remineralize, sealing what were once active caries with a glassy finish. One 14-year-old girl completely healed 42 open cavities in 24 teeth by taking capsules of the high-vitamin cod liver oil and Activator X concentrate three times a day for seven months."

"Activator X also influences the composition of saliva. Price found that if he collected the saliva of individuals immune to dental caries and shook it with powdered bone or tooth meal, phosphorus would move from the saliva to the powder; by contrast, if he conducted the same procedure with the saliva of individuals susceptible to dental caries, the phosphorus would move in the opposite direction from the powder to the saliva. Administration of the Activator X concentrate to his patients consistently changed the

chemical behavior of their saliva from phosphorus-accepting to phosphorus-donating. The Activator X concentrate also reduced the bacterial count of their saliva. In a group of six patients, administration of the concentrate reduced the Lactobacillus acidophilus count from 323,000 to 15,000. In one individual, the combination of cod liver oil and Activator X concentrate reduced the L. acidophilus count from 680,000 to 0."

The principal point is that vitamin K2 is implicated in the proper absorption of minerals. Think of it this way: we're rock and tissue. K2 helps calcium and other minerals to go everyplace they should (bones and teeth), and no place they shouldn't (arteries).

My Experience with K-2

In the mid and late 90's when I began to have regular appointments with my dentist and his hygienist. They referred me to a periodontist, a surgeon who specializes in gum issues. Seems I had some "deep pockets," as they call them, towards the back of my molars that could not be reached with normal cleanings.

Never did I stop to wonder how animals in the wild can possibly manage...without regular brushing, flossing, cleanings and . . . dental surgery.

Because I was still struggling along in business, several years away from hitting a stride, I just opted for the cleanings every three months over the surgery that would set me back a few thousand.

In 2001, with things looking up, I went for the dental surgery. It helped. While I still had to use the numbing mouthwash before each cleaning, it was more effective in those deep pocket areas that used to catapult me to the ceiling in pain when the hygienist would probe them with her sharp poker. This went on for years. The surgery was like a reset button. I now had three cleanings per year, and while things were back to reasonable, it was still only a matter of time until such time that surgery is required again. *Wash. Rinse. Repeat.*

And then in 2008, everything changed. I attribute it to both the Paleo diet and K2.

I ordered the butter oil capsules from Green Pastures—Price's original formulation. I got wind of this product in Dr. Stephan Guyenet's original post on Activator X and his follow-up on where to get it. I noticed some improvement over the first several days in the smoothness of my teeth, particularly upon waking in the morning. And I thought, why not go the distance? So, when my first two bottles ran out and I re-ordered again, this time I also got the fermented cod liver oil caps. Two caps per day of each and the measurable results have been nothing short of phenomenal.

Gobsmacking phenomenal!

Now, about 10 years after having gum surgery and several major teeth cleanings per year, I really don't even find a need to brush my teeth very often. I can literally go days and my teeth remain as though they were pearls in an oyster shell and my tongue is the flesh that explores them. And my gums have not the slightest hint of inflammation, swelling, or anything of the sort. It is remarkable.

Aside from the weight loss via Paleo that got me started on this track in the first place: this, of all things, has been the most remarkably significant and easy to verify aspect of the whole deal.

Additional Resources

- My posts at Free the Animal on Vitamin K2

- Vitamin K2 and Massive Reduction in Heart Disease: Leading Edge

- On the Trail of the Elusive X-Factor: A Sixty-Two-Year-Old Mystery Finally Solved

- Cure Tooth Decay

- Vitamin K2 and the Calcium Paradox

Enhance Your Sex Life Without Pills

I'll end this chapter with another medical issue Paleo can help with: penis enlargement. In a word, your penis emerges when you lose fat. Ignore the scams in infomercials on TV and offers for books and useless products on the Internet. You don't need any of it. You simply need to lose the fat.

Think of your abdominal muscles. You have them. You always have. They're there. They're just hidden by fat. Ab exercises alone will certainly tone and strengthen your abs, but you still won't see them until you lose the fat that's keeping them hidden. And no, sorry, but there's no exercise in the world that "turns fat into muscle." Big. Fat. Lie.

Same goes for the penis enlargement scams. The reason so many men find themselves disappointed in the length of their manliness is because over the years, they've allowed a large donut of fat to grow a little each year around the thing. Lose the fat, and you will experience lengthening and consequent enhanced sexual performance.

Become a Hyperink reader. Get a special surprise.

Like the book? Support our author and leave a comment!

IX.

Eat Like A Caveman

What I Mean By Real Food

Now that you're convinced the Paleo lifestyle will help you lose weight, gain strength, and prevent and treat illness, it's time to start eating!

The Paleo way of eating is simple: eat the foods our ancestors ate before the advent of agriculture and the implementation of industrial practices put processed grains on everyone's plates. *Eat Real Food and nothing but Real Food.*

Let's review what I mean by Real Food:

- Meat (including any organ meats you might like)

- Poultry

- Fish and shellfish

- All vegetables, including starchy ones

- All fruits

- Nuts (except peanuts, which are legumes)

- Fats (lard, tallow, butter, ghee, coconut oil, red palm oil, olive oil)

- Dairy (if you aren't lactose intolerant), such as milk, cheese, cottage cheese, and heavy cream

- Herbs and spices of all sorts

Stay away from grain-based products. All of them, except perhaps on a very occasional splurge. Avoid the processed foods in boxes, bags, cans, and bottles. If you asked your ancestors over the last 2–3 million years (save the last 10,000 or so) to go get enough grain to bake a loaf of bread, it would have taken enormous energy expenditure and time to collect even a handful of kernels. Not only was there no mechanization, but no cultivation either. They'd have had to forage wild grasses. It would have been far easier to hunt, trap or fish a high-density, nutritious meal in the form of an animal.

Stay away from all vegetable/grain/seed oils, except olive, coconut, and red palm (no canola, sunflower, safflower, corn, etc). We simply didn't evolve eating polyunsaturated oils in concentration. It's essentially the same issue as with fruit juices. Would you sit down and eat two dozen oranges? Eating the whole fruit (or vegetable) has its own built in *stop* mechanism: the fibrous bulk fills us up before we overload on sugar.

When you start eating primarily fat and protein, your cravings for grains and sugar will ebb and eventually go away entirely. You'll develop a hunger for real food and real food alone, and you'll be able to *go with how you feel as your first and primary authority.* You won't need to read nutritional advice columns or ask your doctor how to lose weight. You'll be losing it, quickly, by eating the food you were born to eat.

How To Cook Paleo

Going on the Paleo lifestyle means you'll want to cook most of your meals yourself. As a general rule, you should avoid eating out as much as possible. Even the nicest restaurants may use ingredients you should be avoiding, like vegetable-based fats, white flour in sauces, and hidden sweeteners.

My brother recently emailed with a problem that may be familiar to you:

"I am not a cook. You want an over/under absorption and recapitalization analysis on revenue of fifty million dollars per month? No problem; I'll have it done in a day or two. Ask me to plan a healthy menu for the next week, and, well, I'll give you a deer in the headlights look. I don't have a clue. Where do I start?"

Make Your Kitchen Paleo

This means throwing out your sugars, syrups, honey, and other sweeteners—or just keep tiny portions of raw organic honey, molasses, or real maple syrup for occasions. Toss your bread, pasta, and flour. Get rid of most prepackaged items and all processed foods —frozen dinners, meal replacement bars, and of course: cookies and chips. A few exceptions to make life easier might be canned tomatoes and tomato sauce, beef and chicken stock, frozen berry medleys, canned tuna, sardines, oysters (either water packed, or olive oil). Of course, it's always best to go fresh, but these represent sensible conveniences.

Now go to the grocery store or farmer's market and stock up on real food:

1. Buy meat of all types. Choose from beef, lamb, pork, venison, and poultry (especially dark meat). Prefer fresh meats over processed meats like bacon, frankfurters, sausages, hot dogs, and so on.

My favorite cuts include:

- Rib-eyes and filets

- Cheap, flavorful cuts like flank steak, hangar, and flap (bavette)

- Beef, pork and lamb roasts of all sorts

- Beef short ribs

- Lamb shanks

- Pork ribs (back and spareribs)

- Many more; the list is endless

2. Spend time in the produce section. Choose broccoli, cauliflower, mustard greens, collard greens, Swiss chard, tomatoes, potatoes, and sweet potatoes. Include salad greens, like:

- Green leaf lettuce

- Butter lettuce

- Romaine

- Arugula

- Baby spinach

- Kale (ounce for ounce, the most nutrient dense vegetable)

- Many more; the list is endless

I like to mix these together and then add crunch in the form of carrots, green cabbage, red cabbage, jicama, green bell peppers, radishes, and celery. Some grocery stores, such as Trader Joe's, sell these salad mixes chopped and prepackaged.

3. Buy strawberries, blueberries, and blackberries. Over the winter, when it's harder to find fresh berries, buy frozen berry mixes to use in smoothies or eat for dessert.

4. Nuts are good, but they are very calorically dense. I like almonds, macadamia, walnuts, Brazil nuts, hazelnuts, and pecans. Remember that peanuts aren't nuts, but legumes. And be careful with nuts. Most have an adverse omega-6 to omega-3 fat ratio, and they are very calorie dense. Rule of thumb: a handful per day. Note that macadamia nuts have the very best fatty acid profile, with almost no omega-6 fats. Hazelnuts are second best.

5. Buy fats. You want lard (but not the kind that's partially hydrogenated), butter, ghee, coconut oil, and olive oil. Save your bacon drippings. Stay away from *Frankenfats,* like vegetable and canola oil. There is one single exception and that's high-oleic sunflower oil. This is a variety that was selectively bred over time such that over 70% of the fat is monounsaturated. There is relatively little omega-6 and as such, it can be safely used in high heat applications.

6. Your dairy products should always be whole fat. Never buy low fat dairy products, and make your milk and cheese as unprocessed as possible. Go for organic or raw whole, non-homogenized milk (if it's available). Concerns about health issues with raw milk are unfounded. Multitudes more are harmed or killed every year as a result of e-coli contamination of meat and leafy vegetables. I am aware of no such reports in connection with any raw milk producer in the US.

7. Stock your spice cabinet. Choose garlic, cumin, paprika, curry powder, chili powder, cayenne, salt, all types of pepper, and cinnamon. I also love to use Thai massaman curry paste for red meat dishes and yellow or green curry paste for poultry and fish dishes. My favorite herbs are parsley, oregano, basil, tarragon, cilantro, chives, and bay leaves. Spices and herbs add valuable nutrients to the Paleo diet.

A Word About Dairy

Many already familiar with the Paleo lifestyle might object that dairy is not a Paleo food. It's unlikely that Paleo people would have had access to cow and sheep milk in the wild, as those products are a consequence of domestication and agriculture. Moreover, lactose tolerance is actually a genetic mutation that probably took place only around 8,000 years ago. Lactose intolerance was the norm before that. It was nature's way of signalling that it's time to wean.

Acknowledged. Dairy is not a true Paleo food, and so consuming it is not in keeping with a strict Paleo regimen. That said, dairy is highly nutritious on many levels—it has to be, since it's designed as the sole source of nutrition for a growing little one. Add to that the nutritional enhancements that come from processing dairy into various other forms like butter, cream, cheese, yogurt, kefir, and other fermented products.

On the other hand, there are potential problems with dairy, particularly in terms of its protein makeup. Dairy contains specific proteins that promote higher insulin levels and other growth factors, again, for obvious reasons.

So it's your call. If it works for you, go for it, keeping it real and sensible. I stick to butter, cream and a little cheese, usually used as more of a spice than a mainstay. In this way, I'm focusing on the fat portion and leaving most of the proteins out. If I have a nice cold glass of raw (non pasteurized, non homogenized) full-fat milk from a grassfed source, I do it as a treat, an infrequent indulgence.

A Note On Grassfed Meat And Organic Produce

I love grassfed meat and use it often. I have a subscription to a "CSA," which stands for Community Supported Agriculture. These are kind of like co-ops for animal products and vegetable products. Typically, you'll get a box with various things each week, driven by season. CSAs for meats typically include purely grassfed local beef, lamb, and pastured pork, as well as eggs. In terms of produce, you'll get organic fruits and vegetables.

Use Google to search for directories for CSAs in your local area. In terms of buying direct from local farms and ranches, EatWild.com has a search engine for locating these resources in the US, Canada, and internationally. And if there's not a CSA in your area, there are a number of ranches that will ship their grassfed and pastured products to you directly.

I encourage the preference for grassfed and pastured animal products for these reasons:

- **It's healthier.** Most also find it tastier when cooked properly.

- **It's more natural.** Cattle, for example, are not evolved to eat corn, barley or soy. They eat grass. Feeding them grains causes digestion issues in the rumen that then must be combated with antibiotics. It's not a stretch to view this practice as inhumane for the animals, particularly when confined to a Concentrated Animal Feeding Operation (CAFO).

- **It's better for the environment.** You don't have to be an "environmentalist" to understand the absurdity of this scenario: plow under forests and prairies, habitat for creatures and critters of all sorts, in order to plant corn and soy to feed the cattle. Why not simply graze the cattle naturally on the grasslands and natural habitat that existed there in the first place?

However, I want to be as inclusive as possible. You can reap the benefits of Paleo by buying food from grocery chains. I also don't want to discourage someone from the Paleo scene because they feel they don't measure up if all they can reasonably source is grain-finished meat due to budget or other considerations. It's a personal choice. Your emphasis should be on getting results first.

In time, though, don't be surprised if you find your priorities beginning to change. For example, rather than trying to find the cheapest food possible and saving your money for the best 70" flat screen TV you can find, you may begin to view what you are putting in your body as the first priority in your budget.

As you see the weight fall off, you might gradually up your game and start exploring farmer's markets and your local ranchers and dairies. Once you know that this is the way you will eat for life, it's pretty easy to make it economical. After all, you no longer have to buy bread, cereal, granola bars, pasta, and cases of soda pop and fruit juices. In terms of nutrient density, *Paleo is cheap compared to the empty, sugar, flour, crap-laden junk in boxes and packages.*

Joining a local chapter of the Weston A. Price Foundation (WAPF) is a great way to learn about local food sources, get deals for members, and become part of a community with others who share your values.

Cavekids and hunger

A parent and reader of my blog emailed with a problem.

"My problem is with my kids. I handle the cravings pretty well, and the kids are compliant with my decision to eliminate grains, sugar and legumes...However, they are constantly hungry (or think they are). We are very fit and genetically thin and muscular. I am 41, 5'10 and 130 lbs. of cavewoman-style muscle, and a certified Yoga instructor. My kids, 11, 10 and 6 have started showing increased muscle definition—not from 'leaning out' or losing what little fat they had to start with—but they are hungry! They are having increased athletic performance, and clothes are getting tighter in places like thighs, biceps and calves. For 'skinny kids' they look absolutely ripped; and so do I, unlike most people in my rural area in 'flyover country.'

"This is not simply 'craving' the junk they were accustomed to...they feel hungry (Paleo, three months now). Is it just a matter of time? We practice about an 80/20 diet, and I allow dairy in addition to meat, veggies, and fruit. What can I do to help them lessen the 'hungry' feeling?

"...It seems that many are paleo for the weight loss benefits, and we are because I wanted to avoid GMO foods; but we were already healthy and not 'grain-dependent' so this is an unexpected complication."

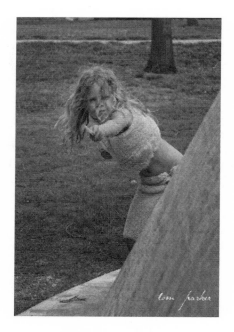

Photo courtesy of Tom Parker

In a subsequent exchange, this reader told me that the kids eat three meals per day, and that they eat a lot, mostly all Paleo foods, but they are still complaining of being hungry all the time.

First and foremost, hunger is a normal evolutionary adaptation to motivate us to source more food, because in the wild, nothing is certain. The problem arises when that survival adaptation is put into a context where we have unlimited supply, and we know it. In the wild, depending on the environment, it's reasonable to assume that where food was relatively accessible, people might choose to tolerate the hunger longer because it's not severe enough to motivate them to go out of their way—kinda like when you delay cooking a meal because it's a chore that's worse than your current level of hunger.

Particularly in the last few decades, we've established as part of our culture the notion that if you're hungry and don't immediately feed, something's wrong, or it's unhealthy, bad for you, etc. Of course, this is the doing of the food conglomerates and their marketing and promotions. We have a food culture that conditions us to never go hungry and never go thirsty, so when you're feeling hungry, go ahead and have that Snickers bar and sugar drink. You'll be hungry again soon enough...

Looking back to my own childhood in the 60s and 70s, I recall how different the food culture was. We had breakfast as a family every morning before anyone left for school or work, and 8-9 times out of 10 it was bacon, eggs, & toast (hash browns were for Sunday breakfast). Rarely did we have oatmeal or boxed cereal. My mom packed a lunch everyday—a sandwich with meat on it, fruit, and usually some carrot sticks or something. A bag of chips was a rare treat and I always envied the other kids who always had them. But what I remember the very most is coming home from school, playing outside (we lived in wide open spaces with huge fields and a river, not a suburban development) for a few hours, coming in and asking mom, "when is dinner; I'm hungry." I can recall the hunger being almost unbearable at times, but having anything to eat was out of the question ("you'll spoil your dinner"). Mom was always a great cook, so I always dug into dinner with gusto. In later years, I recall us being allowed one or two slices of toast with peanut butter in the afternoon. In retrospect, I wish we hadn't been.

Kid hunger is an entirely different animal. Hunger is based on metabolic demands for everyone (in the context of a healthy metabolism); but for kids, this is a moving target on an upward slope. "Eat your food so you can grow up big and strong" is only partially right and implies that it's the food that causes growth. In fact, it's growth hormone that causes growth and hunger and subsequent higher intakes of food is in response to that growth and bigger mass to feed. So, just as growth is not uniform across the life of a child (spurts), so we would expect spurts in severity of hunger and total food intake. Normal.

If you can pack them a *really hearty* Paleo lunch that they can have in lieu of the cafeteria food, I'd do that as absolute step number one. Maybe include an indulgence once per week as motivation. Another motivation, if you have the means, is to sometimes give them plenty to share with friends (make it *good*). If the friends love it and envy them, they're more likely to develop a healthy *elitist attitude*—because, of course, they *are* the elite. That they already demonstrate increased athletic performance at school ties the whole bow on the package.

If milk is part of the dairy they consume, I'd eliminate that and replace it with meat, veggies, fruits, nuts (butter, cream and cheese should be fine).

Involve them in preparation, cooking and cleanup as much as possible. Teach them to begin preparing their own simple dishes. I learned to make simple 2-egg omelets as a kid (plain, or with cheese), I think by about age 9. This will have the effect of putting their hunger into a context: "Hungry means you have to work. Now, how hungry did you say you were?"

And very important, Paleo is not necessarily low carb, regardless of what you may have learned. Paleo includes zero carb to very high carb, depending upon what's available in any given environment. So, don't be afraid of carbs and most particularly so, with kids whose metabolisms should be fine if they're lean and have always been lean. So, get some white sweet potatoes, pierce & pop 'em in the nuker for 5 minutes or so, slit 'em open, spread butter on them and sprinkle with cinnamon. Eat with a spoon. For added delight, toast & caramelize them under the broiler after the butter and cinnamon are added. This could go with a meal, be dessert, or an afternoon snack. I suspect the the addition of some quality carbohydrate in the form of potatoes and fruit will go a long way toward ameliorating their hunger.

Cook plenty at dinner so that there's more than they can possibly eat (and for really good meals, plenty for that lunch to share with friends). Remind them of the hunger they experience and suggest they really make it count. Then if they do get hungry later, let them partake in as much leftovers as they want. Have them get used to eating cold leftovers from the fridge or, make another plate and let it sit out for 30 minutes to get nearer room temperature. This also teaches delayed gratification and, don't be surprised that if they do put the plate out and wait 30 minutes, their appetite might *sometimes* be gone in the interim and the plate goes back in the fridge (happens to me sometimes).

Nothing ever to eat or snack on once dinner is done (this should be near absolute with everyone). This gets their bodies used to going 12 hours per day with nothing but water. I often remark that my intermittent fasting 1-2 times per week for 24-30 hours reset my hunger mechanism to a more normal one, but it's just as likely that a more profound cause is that virtually every day I go about 12 hours minimum without any food or snack. Also, if they complain of hunger a few hours after dinner, before bedtime, have them take note of it and then take note of how hungry they are immediately upon waking. Sleep moderates hunger.

So to summarize, I'd first realize that hunger is normal, and particularly in the context of growing kids where hunger is in part a means of motivating the consumption of more food than they have been accustomed to eating, as they grow. If they're lean as normal kids should be, they have well functioning metabolisms, and now have an opportunity to live their whole lives without ever messing them up. Point out to them all the people who have damaged themselves. You probably have family members like that, where you could show them pictures of what the person looked like in their youth.

So in the context of well functioning metabolisms, let them eat Paleo as much as they want. Just not after dinner. Here's the principle tradeoffs:

1. You get to eat as much Paleo as you want between breakfast and dinner, no limits. In return, nothing between dinner and breakfast.

2. You get to eat Paleo snacks between meals, but you have to do it yourself (leftovers, sweet potato, fruit, etc.) and you have to clean up any mess. (Allowing them such

snacks has the added benefit of likely resulting in additional leftovers from dinner that can be used in lunches.)

3. No more cafeteria food at school, but you get an indulgence once per week, and when there are leftovers from a great dinner, you can have enough to share with friends so they'll envy you, and you can explain how this is why you're so lean & muscular and do better in sports.

Time to Start Cooking

This part is simple, simple, simple. You can teach yourself how to cook through trial and error, which means you'll *really* learn. And the more you teach yourself, the more you learn. Repeat. After all, how do you learn to do anything? You get in and do it, flail and fail, learn, and the process continues.

Use your imagination. Experiment. *Don't be too afraid to ruin something.* Some of the tastiest and easiest preparations include:

- Grilling meats of any kind

- Making meat stews, chili, and curries

- Stir frying veggies

- Making salads with homemade dressing (oil and vinegar, Dijon, etc.)

- Blending cream or coconut milk with egg yolks and berries for a breakfast smoothie

- Soups

The possibilities are truly endless. Turn to the chapter on **"Cold Therapy"** for some examples of Paleo meals.

I don't force myself to be a Paleo "purist." I go out to eat, attend dinner parties at vegetarian friends' houses, and indulge a little during the holidays. But concentrating on real food and passing on processed has resulted in 60 pounds of fat loss, massive reduction in blood pressure, cessation of prescription medications, fabulous lean muscle and strength gains, and a host of other lifestyle improvements.

Eating a Paleo diet is obviously of utmost importance if you want to achieve these results, but the Paleo lifestyle is about more than just food. In the next chapter I'll talk about **fasting** the way our ancestors did to stimulate your metabolism and lose weight fast.

Become a Hyperink reader. Get a special surprise.

Like the book? Support our author and leave a comment!

X.

The Power of Fasting

Intermittent Fasting & Debunking "Several Small Meals A Day"

Over hundreds of thousands of years of evolution, it's only in the last 10,000 years that some people have had the opportunity to never be truly hungry. Wild animals, including wild humans, didn't have pantries and refrigerators, or local supermarkets and restaurants. They had to hunt, gather and prepare their food, and they also had to think and plan for times when food would be scarce. Sometimes they failed.

In short, humans are designed to go significant periods of time without energy intake, and even to expend significant energy (like a hunt, or a chase) prior to being able to eat. Wild animals exist in this fashion. Do wild animals have to eat first or, *is hunting a response to hunger?* The answer seems obvious.

Nutritionally and metabolically speaking, the body can only be in one of two states: fed or fasted. Here's a quote by a popular author on fasting, Brad Pilon. Prior to this, Brad used to be a nutrition researcher for fitness magazines:

". . . the research on weight loss had become so skewed with politics that it has turned into the world's most ironic oxymoron. After all, the research was trying to uncover the completely backwards idea: what should we eat to lose weight?"

When you unpack and unravel everything, it's all fundamentally premised on the same lie: that you must eat, drink, or take something in order to lose fat, and that what you eat, drink, or take is more fundamentally about quality than about quantity. Why? Well, because you can't build a multi billion-dollar "weight-loss" industry on: "don't eat *anything —just don't eat until you're really hungry.*"

Does this sound like it's in conflict with all I've been saying about the Paleo diet? Am I now advocating that you just need to cut the calories? Yes, and no.

The scientific research is pretty clear: in order to lose significant fat, you must operate in a caloric deficit. There's no magic bullet. However, as explained in the **"Fat Is King"** chapter: *all diets are high-fat diets.* You see, you're operating at a caloric deficit only in terms of your food intake. The rest is coming from your own body fat, so you are still in "energy balance." A low- to moderate-carb Paleo diet that reduces baseline insulin levels assists in allowing your cells to release that fat for energy. The result is greater satiation, less appetite, and fat loss.

Intermittent Fasting (IF) simulates the unavailability of food that our ancestors experienced, stimulating the reprogramming of our ancestral appetites and metabolism.

Here's how it works. You already know that a chronically high processed-food diet keeps insulin *chronically* elevated and makes the body gain weight with each passing year, and that eating a predominantly high-fat, low-to-moderate-carb diet (levels determined individually) is one key to keeping your baseline insulin levels down and losing fat. IF also plays a role by helping your body develop **insulin sensitivity,** so that it doesn't keep releasing the extra insulin that your body is used to producing to process sugars. Insulin sensitivity keeps your weight off once you lose it. There's also another hormone called leptin that plays a big role in satiation. In a nutshell, it's a similar thing to insulin. Whereas, with insulin, chronically high levels make people resistant to it, so that the body requires more and more, which tends to keep fat locked in cells chemically. This is why Type 2 diabetics are typically overweight or obese. Similarly, people can become leptin resistant, meaning their brains are no longer hearing the signal that they have enough fat mass and should curtail eating. In fact, obese people have high levels of serum leptin, just as diabetic and pre-diabetics have high serum insulin.

Intermittent Fasting, in combination with eating the Paleo diet, encourages your body to revert to its normal (hunting) weight, making it an important factor in long-term weight loss.

Ignore Advice About Eating Several Small Meals

Mainstream nutritionists and doctors often recommend doing things like eating many small meals per day, never skipping meals, eating a hearty breakfast, making sure to eat before and after a workout, and on and on. Like those who recommend a diet concentrated around whole grains and fruit juices, they're ignoring the lessons we can learn from our ancestors.

Consider this study of alternate day fasting for obese adults:

"To test alternate-day fasting in obese adults, Varady and her colleagues had 12 obese women and 4 obese men begin by eating normally for a two-week control period. Then, for eight weeks, they ate just 25 percent of the calories they needed to maintain their weight, between noon and 2 p.m., every other day."

They ate with no restrictions every over day, and on the fasting days they ate 25% baseline caloric intake in a two-hour feeding window. This was not even a true fast, since they were still eating on the off days, but the results were still still quite impressive:

"Even though the study participants ate whatever they wanted on their non-fasting days, they lost an average of 5.6 kilograms (about 12 pounds) after eight weeks . . .

"People lost anywhere from about 7 pounds to about 30 pounds and that was in a very short amount of time,' Varady said. 'And,' she added, 'the program was pretty easy for the study participants to follow.'"

My own weight loss really accelerated when I incorporated intermittent fasting into my lifestyle. I experienced not only rapid fat loss, but also muscle and strength gains.

The big change came when I incorporated IF into my Paleo and workout plan in late 2007, as I outlined in my first two blog posts on the subject. The first two fasts (right before the holiday break) lost me about a pound. The next two, in the first week of January, lost me about two pounds. But then I began to notice something really interesting and profound: my appetite began to change.

Fasting Changes Your Appetite: Where To Get Started

I started a fasting regimen with 30-hour duration fasts, typically culminating in a 30-minute weight lifting session at the gym. In the months to follow, I lost most of my weight doing 24–30 hour fasts, concluding with a workout. I'd go for 20–28 hours without eating, hit the gym, and then eat big a couple of hours or so after.

Eventually, I gained what I called "high resolution into hunger" by going to the gym, increasing intensity with something like a leg press (heavy weights, large muscle group, and rapid repetitions). Suddenly, I would get very hungry. Then, as I backed off the intensity or finished the set, the hunger would quickly go away. I found I could bring it back and have it go away again, over and over.

This "resolution," or understanding, or enlightenment with regard to hunger, meant that my hunger was no longer tied to the clock. I could be hungry at any given time or satiated at any given time, irrespective of traditional "meal times."

Then I understood why my two dogs, who have been on an evolutionarily appropriate diet for some time, didn't seem to care about meal times. I understood why they would intermittently pass up food, even when it was sitting in front of them, or, at times, be insatiable no matter what.

Ever pigged out on a pizza or an enormous plate of spaghetti until you felt as though you'd pop, and couldn't imagine ever eating again for the rest of your life? And then, mysteriously, did you feel hungry again in only a few hours? Did you stop to note that perhaps the hormonal signals regulating your hunger and satiation are completely screwed up? It's because they are. Most people eat modern processed food diets and never allow themselves to go hungry for any appreciable amount of time.

Since losing the weight, I have gone to a far more intermittent model. Sometimes I just skip meals, and I don't eat when I'm not really hungry. Sometimes I'll go for 12 hours, sometimes 20 or more. The Paleo model, combined with IF, has reset me to a more natural state. I can truly rely on my hunger to tell me when my body needs food.

Fasting also heightens the senses and stimulates heightened cognitive function. The evolutionary logic for that claim should be obvious: for survival's sake, you need to be at your best when it's on the line. Most studies I've seen don't support my claim, but this has been my experience and that of many others who've commented on my blog and elsewhere.

Are we all just fooling ourselves, or is there a logical explanation? I think there is. All the studies include people who've likely *never fasted or gone hungry for any significant period of time in their lives.* Regular IFers adapt to fasting over time, resetting themselves to a natural state. We're accustomed to fasting as nature intended.

How To Start Fasting

Depending on your age, you've likely been feeding regularly and continuously for decades, day in and day out. Your body isn't even aware that it can go months without anything but water. In a sense, eating three meals a day with snacks in between isn't much different from any other kind of addiction. At first, fasting feels like getting off caffeine, nicotine, alcohol, and other drugs your body may have become comfortably accustomed to. Your body is going to put up a big fuss when denied. *It won't be easy, but it's worth the results.*

To make a 24–36 hour fast as easy as possible, follow these steps:

1. Have your last meal around 3–4 p.m. initially. Then go to bed that night, sleep like a baby, get up at 6 or 7 a.m., and your body will have prepared you for fasting during sleep by releasing hGH. By now you're already at 18 hours.

2. The next day, keep yourself busy until dinner. You can break your fast around 7 p.m. or later, depending on how long you wish to extend it. When you get really hungry, get really busy, or, depending on your personal circumstances, take a nap.

3. If possible, get in a workout early afternoon. This should be around the 22–24 hour mark. If you get your intensity up (with a lot of weight), it will kill your hunger for a few hours. What I've found, however, is that the hunger that returns in the later afternoon is of a very pleasant and warm kind. That signals that you've broken through, and your body has adapted to the fast and is easily releasing enough fat to keep your energy levels up and your hunger at bay.

4. Break your fast with meat, potatoes, fruit and other Paleo food. Eat big. Some people develop problems with fasting because it can become a rather euphoric experience, and so they gradually slide into either fasting too often or not eating sufficiently when they're not fasting. If you're past the point of needing to lose weight, *then you should view a fast as simply postponing eating, not eating less.* You're merely crowding what you would normally eat in seven days, into into five or six days. Additionally, if you're approaching this from a low to moderate carbohydrate perspective, then post-workout and breaking a fast are the times to load up on whole food carbohydrates like potato, sweet potato and fruit. This restores glycogen stores to the liver and muscles.

Fasting For Cleansing: Autophagy

Just like the rather silly notion of "what do I eat to lose weight?" there is the equally silly notion of "what do I eat to cleanse?" In fact, fasting is the only valid cleansing mechanism. It gives your system a rest, allows your bacterial gut flora to readjust to normal proportions and even cleanses on a cellular level through a process known as autophagy, or "self eating." From Wikipedia:

"In cell biology, autophagy, or autophagocytosis, is a catabolic process involving the degradation of a cell's own components through the lysosomal machinery. It is a tightly regulated process that plays a normal part in cell growth, development, and homeostasis, helping to maintain a balance between the synthesis, degradation, and subsequent recycling of cellular products. It is a major mechanism by which a starving cell reallocates nutrients from unnecessary processes to more-essential processes.

"A variety of autophagic processes exist, all having in common the degradation of intracellular components via the lysosome. The most well-known mechanism of autophagy involves the formation of a membrane around a targeted region of the cell, separating the contents from the rest of the cytoplasm. The resultant vesicle then fuses with a lysosome and subsequently degrades the contents.

"It was first described in the 1960s, but many questions about the actual processes and mechanisms involved still remain to be elucidated. Its role in disease is not well categorized; it may help to prevent or halt the progression of some diseases such as some types of neurodegeneration and cancer, and play a protective role against infection by intracellular pathogens; however, in some situations, it may actually contribute to the development of a disease."

What this all means is that when you fast for more extended periods, your cells clean out and recycle your intracellular garbage.

There is new research being conducted having to do with starving cancer cells through fasting. Cancer cells can only utilize glucose, and not glycogen or ketone bodies. Moreover, cancer cells are 20–30 times less efficient at glucose utilization than normal cells. Cancer cells are real sugar addicts.

There is also research on fasting as a way to mitigate the harmful effects of chemotherapy. Chemo is equally toxic to healthy cells as it is to cancer cells. Chemo is a war of attrition, in which one hopes to kill the cancer before killing the host. But not if the healthy cells and the cancer cells have undergone a prolonged fast prior to undergoing chemo. Researchers have demonstrated that fasting prior to chemo puts healthy cells into a protective posture (and perhaps compromises cancer cells due to the lack of dietary sugar) and changes the game from 1-to-1 attrition, to one of an important advantageous "kill ratio" of cancer cells to healthy cells.

I also cited this report in a post at Free the Animal:

"During the study, conducted both at USC and in the laboratory of Lizzia Raffaghello at Gaslini Children's Hospital in Genoa, Italy, the researchers found that current chemotherapy drugs kill as many healthy mammalian cells as cancer cells.

"'(But) we reached a two to five-fold difference between normal and cancer cells, including human cells in culture. More importantly, we consistently showed that mice were highly protected while cancer cells remained sensitive,' Longo said.

"If healthy human cells were just twice as resistant as cancer cells, oncologists could increase the dose or frequency of chemotherapy.

"'We were able to reach a 1,000-fold differential resistance using a tumor model in baker's yeast. If we get to just a 10–20 fold differential toxicity with human metastatic cancers, all of a sudden it's a completely different game against cancer,' Longo said."

I don't claim fasting will be easy the first, second, or even third time, but just like anything else, you get good at it and it becomes a familiar path. We've got millions of years of evolutionary adaptation that says our bodies are built for survival in very sparse and inhospitable conditions. The human species would not have survived the mass migration to populate the entire globe, from equator to arctic and sea level to 16,000 feet, otherwise. The ability is baked into our genome.

Fasting is the path to expressing those long dormant genes, and you will not believe how it will *Free the Animal* in you—and by this I mean a languid, content, focused animal, one completely free of rage, frustration, and other unhealthy toxins.

Additional Resources

- Posts at Free the Animal on fasting

- EatStopEat

- Fast5

- Leangains

Become a Hyperink reader. Get a special surprise.

Like the book? Support our author and leave a comment!

XI.

Evolutionary Exercise And Fitness

The 1-Hour Per Week Workout Regimen

When exercise and working out comes up in conversations, I like to challenge people to guess how much time I spend at the gym. Hours per week, they think. They're always surprised to hear the truth: *I go to the gym for one hour per week—never, ever, more.* I split that hour into two sessions per week. Every few months I take a week off.

Back when I started on my path to weight loss, I thought walking 3-plus miles per day was the way to go. In five to six years and 5,000–6,000 miles, I put on another 25 pounds instead of losing weight. Walking just made me hungrier, and I'd come home and eat like I'd just won something. My finely tuned fat-storing machine was all too happy to gobble up those calories and convert them to more fat.

When I combined the workouts with a more evolutionary approach to eating, I was able to get the ball rolling to more rapid fat loss. And then adding the IF, as discussed in the **"Eat Like A Caveman"** chapter, supercharged the progress.

Now my routine is constructed to *roughly simulate* the activity my ancestors would have received. I take one or two 20-minute walks every day with my dogs. I visit the gym to push, pull, and lift heavy things one to two times per week, 20–30 minutes per session. I do three to six, 15–30 second sprints—or intervals on a stationary bike—once per week.

That's all.

Cardio

If you love it, which would be hard to believe, then knock yourself out. If it's not excruciatingly boring, which would be hard to believe, then knock yourself out. If you enjoy an exhilarating jog or run in cool, misty weather, as I used to do when I lived in the Pacific northwest, then go for it. If you hate running in the humid air of the southeast, or the arid oven of Arizona, then why do it?

As it was for everything else our ancestors experienced, environment and circumstances vary and are different around the world. And your response to those environmental conditions would vary equally.

We're not the equivalent of a diesel generator running in some basement at a constant RPM for hours or days on end. Rather, we're adaptive beings, explosive beings, languishing beings. Arthur De Vany, in his essay on Evolutionary Fitness that "started it all," said it best:

"The adaptive and variable energy demands of our ancestral existence are gone. We live a low energy flux and metabolically unvaried existence in bodies designed for another lifeway. We are hunter/gatherers in pin-stripe suits, living a sedentary life and it is killing us in ways our ancestors never experienced. Virtually all the degenerative diseases—atherosclerosis, diabetes, high blood pressure, and osteoporosis, declining muscle mass—of modern civilization are unheard of among hunter-gatherers and were not part of our ancestral experience.

"Most modern fitness prescriptions are static and agricultural. These programs model the body as a machine, not as an adaptive organism. Consequently, they prescribe a regime in which the body is underfed and over-trained. They are not based on adaptation, but on steady state analysis. These models assume the body is a linear process that maintains a steady state. In fact, all bodily processes are highly non-linear and these non-linearities must be exploited in any effective fitness program. The key to exploiting the highly non-linear and dynamic adaptive metabolic processes of the human body is to achieve the right mixture of intensity and variety of activities."

To Work Out

Depending upon your personal preferences and goals, there are a number of different techniques or methods you can employ. Unless you have specific goals of extreme abs-ripped leanness combined with superhuman strength, you probably don't need to stress about it. Just follow some principles.

Cardio is catabolic, which means that it wastes lean tissue (and makes you hungry). Compare an Olympic sprinter with a marathoner.

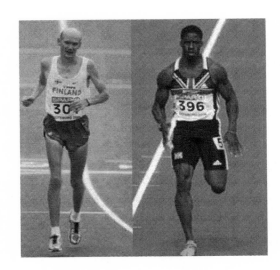

If you do go to the gym and have been for some time, think back. Look at the body compositions on those people you've seen on the treadmill, elliptical and other such torture machines day in, day out, going back years. How much has their body composition improved in that time? Conversely, check out the weight room, where you're likely to have observed some progress.

The principle that matters most to me is *compound movement*. What do I mean? Well, compare the act of taking a dumbbell and doing single arm curls with that of hauling a dead animal carcass back to camp.

I focus on simple, classic lifts that are compound in nature, employing *systems* of compound muscle engagement, usually with free weights in preference to machines:

- Deadlifts

- Squats (back, front, air, etc.)

- Leg presses (typically as a substitution for pure squats)

- Bench presses (careful with the rotator cuffs; these should not be done heavy unless you are very experienced or you have professional training consultation)

- Standing overhead presses

- Weighted chin-ups or pull-ups (you can use a machine at first that will lower your body weight, then get to your body weight, and gradually add weight on a belt)

Really, the above is all anyone ever needs, provided you get to a point where weight is really heavy, by which I mean one to two sets and no more than 10 reps per set. In other words, you find the weight per exercise where you *can't* do more than that.

As an example, the deadlift is my favorite exercise of all, and from the age of 49–50, I began at of a level of about 165 pounds in two sets, five repetitions each. Shortly before my 50th birthday, I had built up to four reps at 305 pounds, and a second set of 275 pounds for four repetitions. Here's a two-minute video of that. I subsequently reached 325 pounds for that lift in five repetitions.

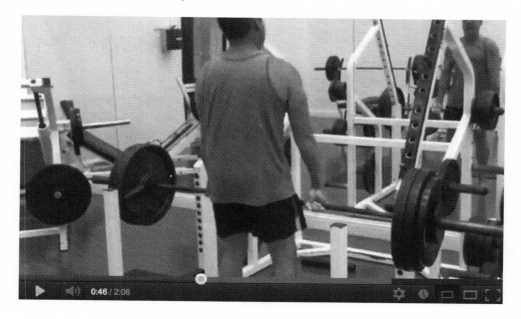

Deadlifts at 305 pounds 4 repetitions

But I was going for a specific goal, and you may not be. More importantly, you don't need to be. So let's cover a few simple bodyweight exercises:

- Push ups (the king; and you can begin with incline, go flat, and then step it up with decline)

- Pull ups or Chin ups

- Air Squats (otherwise known as "deep knee bends")

There are also plyometrics, Crossfit, and combinations of those. For all of the foregoing lifts and movements, I encourage you to go to Google or YouTube and simply plug in the movement terms that are unfamiliar to you. There's a plethora of both textual explanations of proper form and procedures, as well as video demonstrations of how to perform the moves properly so as to avoid injury. Have some fun.

Girls and women afraid to lift weights for fear of bulking their muscles: **you're not going**

to "bulk up." Stop using that silly excuse not to lift. However, *you can still be strong even if you aren't bulked.* Remember me beating my chest about a 305 and then 325-pound deadlift, above? Well, here's a not bulked girl pulling 370 pounds. Watch it. Now, that's a 1RM or, one rep max. She's not going to be doing a number of reps at that weight, but neither, obviously, is she pumped up on steroids, nor is she "bulked."

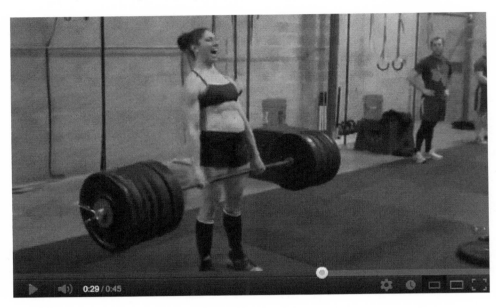

Laura DeMarco deadlift, 370 pounds 1 repetition

Make it count when you hit the gym. An hour per week, two sessions: that's all. *Make it count.*

Kettle Bells

While I've done some form of resistance training all along, and even the Leangains protocol, I'd never done much but some kettlebell swings and presses at the gym I used to go to. Now, I have these in my backyard. In pounds, they're 26, 35, and 44. I've been advised to add a 53.

Mostly, I'd initially just been having fun with them in a totally random fashion almost daily. Could be for a couple of minutes, or 5, or 10. Little to no structure. You can go to YouTube, search, and see any number of exercises performed. You can also find classes in your local area. Kettlebells provide a very flexible but effective way to work out that's nothing like dumbbell curls at the gym, not the intensity of deadlifts and squats, but something in-between many might find to hit their sweet spot as their primary or sole workout regimen or like me: heavy in the gym every week once or twice, fun with kettlebells at random.

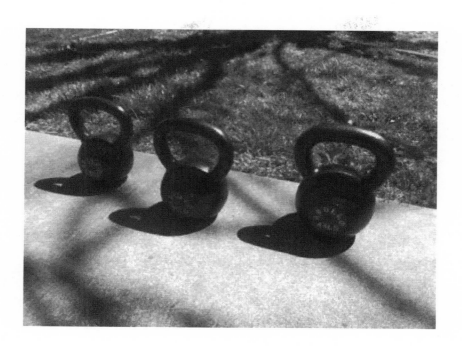

Friends

For more on kettlebells and two different perspectives, see a guest post at my blog by an amateur plugging his way through, and a recent visit to my backyard by a kettlebell expert, Clifton Harski.

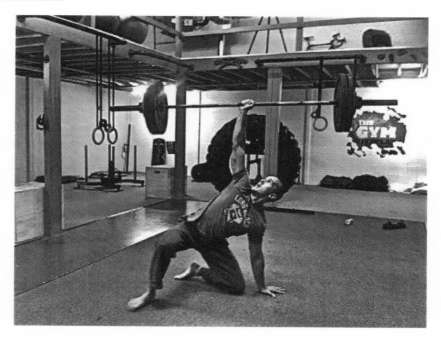

Clifton Harski

A list of kettlebell exercises to search on Google & YouTube for proper procedure and form:

- Bottom up rack walk

- Farmer carry

- Suitcase deadlift

- Single leg deadlift

- Goblet squats

- Single side front squat

- Reverse lunge

- Turkish get up (the Holy Grail)

- RKC swings

- Windmill

- Standing press

- Halo

- Rows

- Floor press

Live Shamelessly

Committing yourself to some manner of flexible workout routines described above is an excellent way to enhance your loss of weight while protecting and even gaining muscle in the process. Imagine living in a time when humans depended on their strength and endurance to meet their basic survival needs. *Imagine having a body that could sprint, hunt, and play.*

Part of the joy of the Paleo lifestyle is regaining the ability to use your body as you did when you were a child. When the weight starts coming off and you feel your muscles getting stronger (often, they'll let you know without any prompting), you'll have the urge to take up former passions you may have abandoned because of weight, age, poor health, and diminished strength.

I've always been adventurous and risk taking, and some years back, I took up the sport of hang gliding. It's a difficult sport to master, as it requires both strength and a measure of endurance. I was able to solo in powered aircraft inside of a couple of months, but it took months of hard effort to get anywhere close in a hang glider.

Hang gliding can be scary at times, due to unpredictable weather conditions, unfamiliarity with where you're launching, flying, and landing, and other factors. Of course, this is an enormous aspect of the allure. I can remember months from those early years during which I thought of little else besides flying.

That was before McDonald's and pizza had their way with me. It wasn't possible to keep flying after I'd put on so much weight.

When I started living Paleo, I lost enough weight to start flying again, and more importantly, to have the *passion* to start flying again. I'm leaner and stronger than I've ever been. Now flying is less chore, more pleasure. I've regained the requisite confidence. It has reawakened me, and I hold Paleo eating, going hungry now and then, and lifting heavy weights responsible.

Here's a couple of short videos that might give you insight into this particular passion of mine I rediscovered, the beginning and end of 30–40 minute flights: here and here. Or, if you're reading on a capable device, here are the videos in sequence.

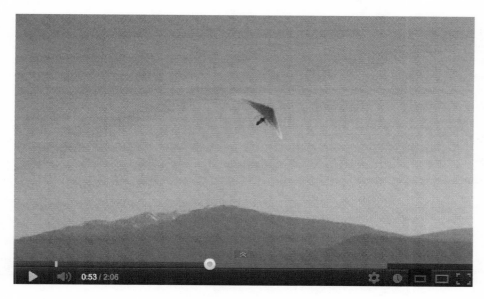

2-minute clips of a 40-minute flight, Hat Creek Rim

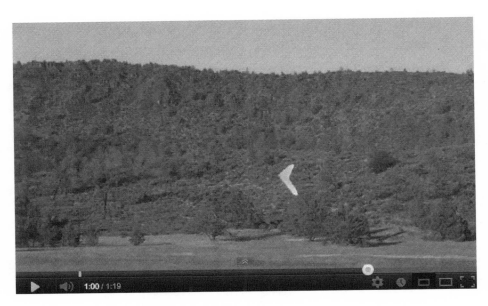

Launch & landing of a 30-minute flight, Hat Creek Rim

How or what do you "fly"? Can you think of something that was once a passion that went by the wayside when you got heavy, old, unhealthy, or some combination thereof?

Go Paleo and you can do it again!

Become a Hyperink reader. Get a special surprise.

Like the book? Support our author and leave a comment!

XII.

Cold Therapy

Cold thermogenesis, or cold therapy, has the power to take you from someone who absolutely must be warm and cozy at all times to someone who can go shirtless in the cold, if you dare. Basically, the idea is to get yourself to adapt to cold over time using either cold air or immersion in very cold water for a time. I caution against packing in ice. Water is far different. There's no risk of frostbite or local nerve damage from freezing a small part of you

Sounds crazy, right? I call it the reset button. I'll explain. But if my explanation completely fails you, I'll give you a pass at the end.

I started cold therapy in 2007 at my gym. It was less than a 5 minute walk away, and it had a "cold plunge" they kept at around 45 deg F. My routine was to workout, get in the sauna for 10 minutes, steam room for a few, jacuzzi for a few, then into the ice water. Initially, 30 seconds was all I could bear, but I found myself totally rejuvenated. Over time, I found I needed more time to get that feeling. Soon I was sitting in there for 3 minutes, then 5. By the time I moved away over a year ago, I was usually soaking for 12-15 minutes after every workout, and I'd occasionally sneak away from home for a fix on the side.

Alright, the above is a bit tongue in cheek, but there's a meaningful thread to it. That is, as unpleasant as it was, *I could never not do it.* And at times, even when I dreaded what I knew was going to happen, and I'd say to myself, "ok, but only for 3 minutes," I'd end up breaking a time record.

I liked it so much I eventually got a big plastic tub for the backyard, the sort of thing they use to water livestock. I'd fill it with the garden hose and except in the summertime, the water is usually 50-55 deg F. I started doing it every day, staying in for as little as 15 minutes and as long as 35 with the average probably falling in the 20-25 minute range. I was not aiming for any specific results, but rather to simply get used to doing it nearly every day and making it a habit that I'd enjoy.

I have obtained one very specific result. I'm a bit hypothyroid and have been for years, with elevated TSH, low normal range for both T3 and T4. The only symptom I suffer that I'm aware of is cold hands and feet, sometimes. Well, and this was pretty amazing, but from *my very first session* almost a month ago, 26 minutes at 52 degrees, I have not experienced cold hands or feet a single time. Not once. In fact, I sometimes feel as though I'm radiating heat off the palms of my hands and soles of my feet. Weird.

Other results include phenomenal sleep and a general sense of having a far wider comfort zone for whatever the ambient temperature is. I'm comfortable when it's 60 deg in the house when I get up, and comfortable now, when it's 77 inside the house. And I didn't even know it got up to 90 outside today until I saw the temp while in my car.

The strangest, most counter-intuitive thing I've experienced, however, is this: *60 degree water is "colder" than 50 degree water.* Of course, what I mean by that is it *feels* colder and I feel colder faster, shiver sooner. At 50 degrees, I have no problem staying in for 30 minutes, feel warm for the first 10 minutes, and don't begin feeling really cold until about the 20-minute mark. At 60 degrees I began feeling really cold in the 10-15 minute range and at 20 minutes, I'm really itching to get out. My speculation is that 50, and perhaps even down to 40 (which I used to do at the gym), is a "sweet spot" where your body mounts a bigger defensive response in preserving blood at your core and thus doesn't feel as cold as quickly as 60. The takeaway for those experimenting with this—dipping their toe in the water as it were—is if you don't get the water down to 50, you may feel as though you can't adapt, and give up.

My own backyard cold plunge.

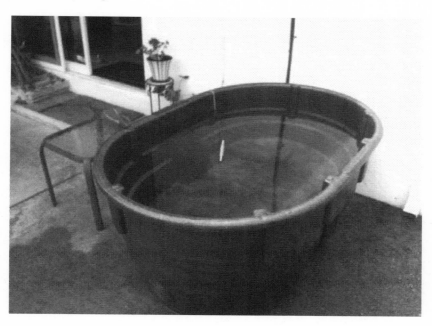

It's a 150 gallon livestock watering trough made by Rubbermaid. I bought this at a local feed and supply place for about $200.

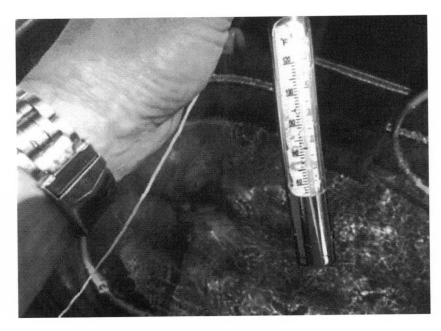

50 degrees, as it's filling

And then, I couldn't wait any longer, and I got right in.

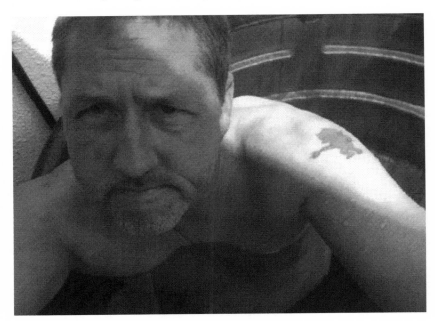

The first time I stepped into the tub, I was filled with horror. This isn't going to be fun! But I just sank right down, the trough overflowed to the point where I could sit, feet exactly touching the other side, and the water comes up to my chin. It's like this was designed to my own bodily specs.

Within 30 seconds I was totally fine, and by 1 minute, actually warm and didn't feel cold until well after 10 minutes. Slight quivers began at the 20-minute mark.

. . . OK, so if you didn't know it by now, it's confirmed: I'm certifiable—and I don't even have a chapter on walking barefoot as most everywhere one can. Here's the deal: I want to give you everything I've found beneficial for me, but it's not necessary to go much beyond the dietary aspects, which are at least 80% of the whole deal. Fasting is a plus. Working out is a plus. A number of things are a plus, including cold adaptation but let me make this very clear: *EVERYTHING BEYOND THE DIET IS MORE VARIABLE, INDIVIDUAL AND ABOVE ALL . . . OPTIONAL!*

That said, let's take a look at what a NASA scientist discovered about cold adaptation and fat loss. Ray Cronise got fat himself, to the tune of 50 pounds over—pretty much like me. He heard that Olympic Athlete and Gold Medalist Michael Phelps eats 12,000 calories per day. It didn't make sense to him that his training load (physical exertion) could account for nearly that.

He had an epiphany.

He hypothesized that because of the thermal conductivity of water vs. air is 24 times as great, that if you spend 15 minutes in very cold water, it's like adding minutes of caloric burn to your day without actually adding minutes. The key is: not to eat more. Or, much more.

Because of the nature of Ray's discovery, he was invited to speak at TEDMED in 2010.

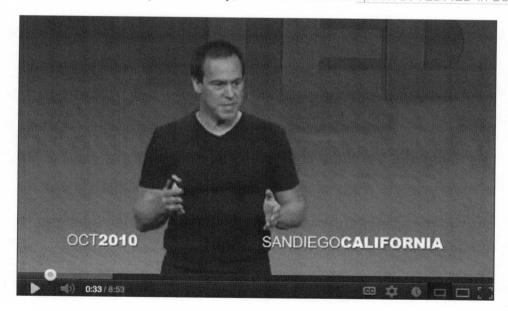

Ray Cronise – TEDMED – on Cold Therapy

Essentially, he was able to dramatically increase the rate of weight loss up to 4 pounds per week, the important thing being that he sees the results he wants sooner and quicker, making it that much more likely that he'll stick with it. And he did.

But again, this is not an essential aspect of anything Paleo or what this book is primarily about, which is: the food. Use whatever you like, as you like.

And finally there's nothing magical or spooky about this as I explain in this video while actually in the tub.

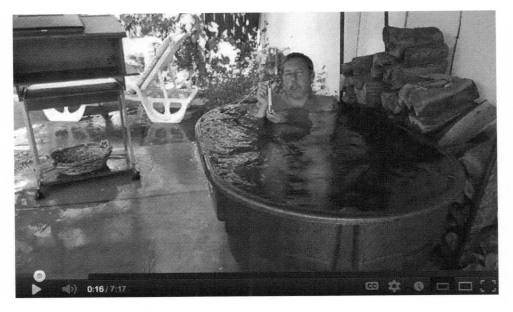

Cold Water Therapy, Thermogenesis, or Exercise

Become a Hyperink reader. Get a special surprise.

Like the book? Support our author and leave a comment!

XIII.

A Primal Weight Loss and Health Improvement Plan

Weight Loss Regimen With The Paleo Plan

The whole weight loss industry is run like a religion. It operates by making you feel guilty for your own nature. And when you feel guilty, you are susceptible to all manner of suggestion—like purchasing ineffective products and services, and punishing yourself with boring diets and hunger-inducing workouts.

Drop the guilt, first and foremost. You've been lied to. You've been told to eat in a manner and exercise in a manner that sets up hormonal cascades guaranteed to leave you forever ravenous and result in muscle loss and fat gain. You can't even believe you've gained this weight, and why? *Because you can look back and recall that you were hungry all the time.* Weren't you? And you were all the more tempted to eat, thanks to that old, familiar paradigm of the "forbidden fruit," making "cheating" all the more enticing.

Leave Original Sin to the religious. You are simply not responsible for feeling hungry, and you can hardly be expected, long term, to ignore and deny those feelings. Hunger always wins.

What you need is a proper diet that satisfies you, and you need an activity and exercise regimen that fills you with playful exuberance. Here's a short plan you can print out and carry around with you:

1. **Try to eat as much as a gram of protein per day per pound of ideal body weight.** This will be about 150–200 grams for the average male, 100–150 for the average female. Be intermittent, as though the food is seasonal, just like hunting.

2. **Eat more fat.** In fact, 50% to 65% of your energy could or should be coming from fat, natural fat: lard, butter, tallow, ghee, coconut oil, olive oil, red palm oil . . . not to mention the fat content of your Real Foods. Stay away from all others to reduce pro-inflammatory omega-6 fats, and take about one to two grams of fish oil per day in order to further get your omega 6 and 3 ratio to a natural, near 1:1 as possible. Eat as much of these fats as you want, as often as you want (except the fish oil).

3. **Eat natural carbohydrates only: veggies, fruits, nuts, tubers, and sweet potatoes.** Eat as many veggies as you want, but be sensible about fruit—a few pieces per day should be fine. No processed food at all. No neolithic foods like grains, corn, legumes; dairy in moderation, if at all. Carbohydrate sensitivity is highly varied individually. If you're already fat, chances are you'll need to avoid potatoes and other natural carbs, because your natural satiation point is out of whack. If not, you may be able to enjoy them, but stick to carbs that come in natural, starchy packages. You have to find this out for yourself.

4. **Don't use any artificial sweeteners or eat anything with artificial sweeteners.** Abstaining from them for a time will help reset your taste to a natural one.

5. **Drop the cardio completely.** Walk outside if you like, as much as you want, and then do full-body resistance workouts twice per week, 30 minutes each, *and go all in every time*. Intensity is the key. For twice a week, 20–30 minutes, you can get intense. Do a few sprints instead of cardio but be careful with sprints, especially if not accustomed to running. Start at a jog and slowly build up speed. Don't be explosive off the line, as this is where most injuries occur.

6. **Select a weight for each exercise such that you can do 6-8 reps in 2 sets.** Get some rest in-between sets, as with higher volume, you want to attack each time. Whenever you can comfortably do 8-9 reps in both sets, increase the weight 5-10% the next time. Progress slowly.

7. **Do full body every time, and focus on legs, chest, back, and shoulders.** Forget arms and abs, and isolation moves in general. These others, especially legs, are the bigger muscles that will stimulate hGH release when loaded significantly. Do deadlifts, standing presses, squats (or leg presses), weighted chin-ups and bench press (not too heavy, protect your shoulders).

8. **Eat two to three times per day on days you eat, or, eat once some days, three times others, two times still others, and nothing now and then.** This models nature and begins turning on dormant genes that want to you be lean and young.

9. **Begin rehabilitating your broken hunger mechanism with one to two fasts per week.** Start with fasts that last 24–30 hours each, and consume only water, unsweetened coffee, or tea. Once you get used to this (three to four fasts), then

arrange it so you're doing your workout at at least 22 hours into the fast. Do animals hunt on full bellies? Don't eat until at least an hour or two after completing a workout.

10. **Get lots of sleep.** Sleep promotes hGH release.

11. **Be cold sometimes.**

And there you have it: eleven simple, fun, natural, sustainable-for-life steps that will work for good, guaranteed.

A Little Heads Up For Beginners

Let me give give you a brief list of things to look out for, so that you don't get discouraged. Expect these things to happen. If they don't, great. If they do, you saw 'em coming.

1. **Ever heard of "hitting the wall?"** It's a term long-distance and marathon runners use to describe glycogen (stored carbohydrate) depletion. When that happens, your body has to convert to lipolysis (fat burning). This is where you want to be—not all the time, but evolution suggests that our primitive ancestors spent much time in this state. Getting through that wall the first time, especially if you've been a big carb muncher, can be tough on some. You might experience days on end of lethargy. *Persist.*

2. **Given #1, I recommend just getting it over with.** This is one area where a the Atkins diet has a real benefit, with its two-week induction of near zero carbohydrate. It makes the unpleasantness of getting used to being a steady fat burner quick. Add in a couple sessions per week of high-intensity resistance training of about 30 minutes, and you'll get your glycogen transport system at attention and get your body adapted to lipolysis all the quicker.

3. **You might experience constipation.** People will tell you to take psyllium husks and such, but my advice is to up the fat content. It's quite lubricative. I recommend more fat because I don't think you should get yourself relying on an unnatural substance. Your body will adapt soon enough.

4. **Most of the initial weight loss is water.** Stored glycogen requires water. For every gram of glycogen, you retain 2.5-3 grams of water, and as you expend the glycogen, you release water. Once you start having to relieve yourself every hour for a couple of days, you'll know you're on the right track. You're going to see an initial big weight drop that's mostly water, then it's going to slow. Don't get discouraged.

5. **Finally, if you get the weight training intensity where it should be, you may gain some weight at first.** Expect it. Embrace it. You're building muscle, which is more dense than fat. Over time, you'll see that you'll have bursts of fat loss to the downside, and bursts of muscle gain to the upside. Eat right, and you'll have more downward bursts over time, and the fat will come off.

And be careful out there. You do yourself no good if you injure yourself right from the start. It's not a race. It's a Life Way.

Become a Hyperink reader. Get a special surprise.

Like the book? Support our author and leave a comment!

XIV.

Recipes And Supplements

Recipes to Complement The Paleo Diet

As I mentioned in the **"Eat Like A Caveman"** chapter, you learn how to cook exactly like you learned everything else you've ever set out to do in life: *you just do it*. There is nothing holding you back besides fear of potential embarrassment or waste. Dismiss both of these worries. Only cook for guests those dishes you've mastered. And how much gas do you waste, ever? Just get over your fears and let yourself experiment.

You can watch cooking shows on TV, or buy cookbooks or Google recipes to get started. Do whatever suits you, but nothing will really compare to just diving right in and learning, failing, correcting, improving, and repeating.

Here are some *random* approaches to breakfast, lunch, and dinner. It's difficult to provide a detailed meal plan, because I never eat in any formula, and I rarely prepare meals by a single recipe. I'm more inclined to use Google to find several recipes and then create my own from ideas I like in several recipes rather than furnishing some solid road map so that you can just do what I say. I want to encourage you to think for yourselves, as though your life depended upon it—which, incidentally, it does. These are just examples. Nothing more.

Breakfast is typically and traditionally some form of egg, some meat, perhaps potatoes, fruit, and so on. You can also think outside the box. Ever eaten leftover meat, veggies and/or salad in the morning? That's an option too. They can be eaten for lunch as well. My main focus is to give you ideas and inspiration; but in fact, all of these dishes can be eaten anytime you like. This goes for all meals. In some cases, I'll give you a link to a specific blog post so you can go get my own recipe. But in most cases, recipes are beyond the scope of this book because I want you to start thinking for yourself. Real food: get it and cook it, because you can, and you should. These are just examples of what I did once I decided to shop real food and cook it for myself.

Every single one of these plates represent ingredients I sources locally and prepared at home. I hope you understand and appreciate it, because it's how I generally eat almost every day.

And remember: you can learn all you need to know in a few minutes by going to Google for every term or recipe you are unfamiliar with.

The following examples are all completely or closely "Paleo." In a few cases there is a grain indulgence (1/2 flour tortilla), some white rice, and dairy.

"Breakfast"

Some Egg, Meat and Fruit Examples

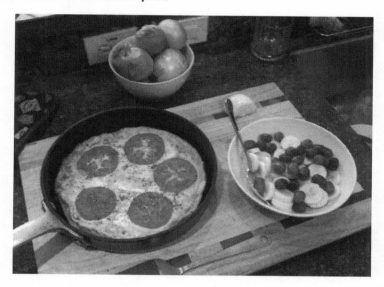

Frittata with mixed fruit

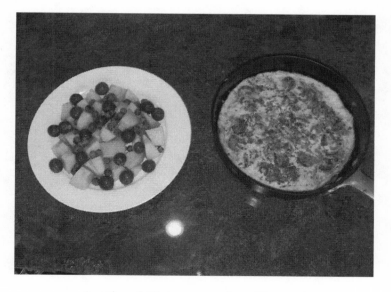

Another frittata example, with meat

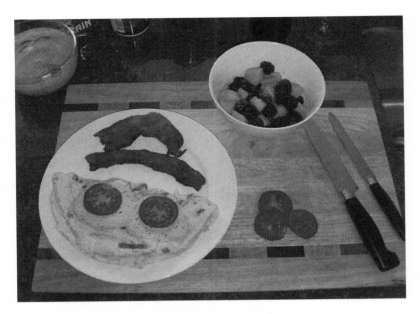

An omelet with creme fraiche sauce, bacon and fruit (Recipe)

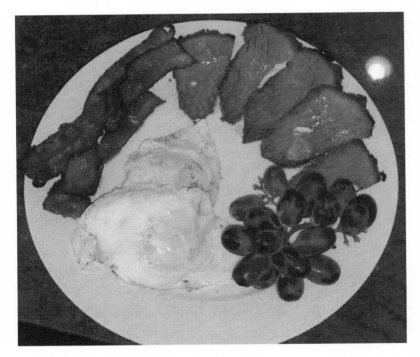

Over easy eggs cooked in butter, bacon, leftover meat and a bit of fruit

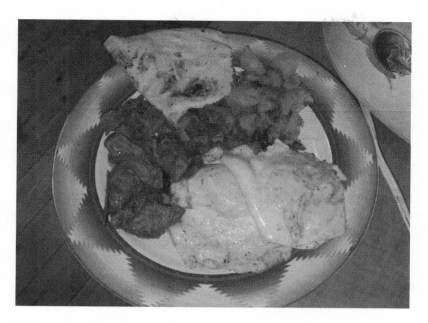

Chili verde with eggs and a ½ flour tortilla indulgence (Recipe)

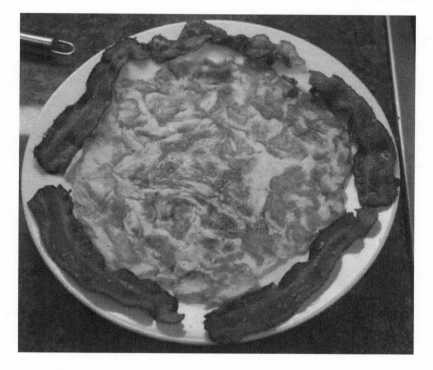

Simple plain omelet cooked in butter, with bacon

Some Classic "Lunch" Ideas

Again, a great strategy is to spend your biggest effort making a dinner you plan and are proud of, but to do enough that you and family can eat leftovers for lunch or even breakfast the next day. This will make things so much easier for you. Then do the fancy breakfast frittatas on the weekend.

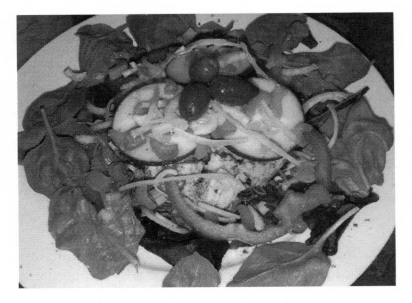

A "Big Salad" with spinach and tuna

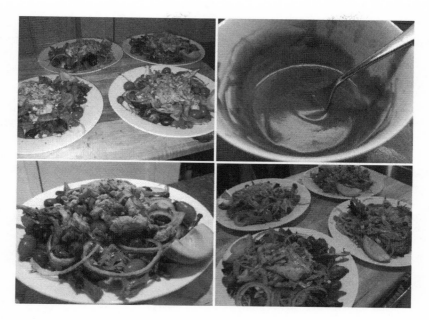

Just another big salad with tuna or chicken, and a dijon vinaigrette

Dinners and Making Enough for Leftovers

It would be great to really use your time, effort and money to plan out and go all out for dinner, for you and your family. And since you're already involved, why not make enough for the next day? Some dishes work better for that than others, but you can figure that out.

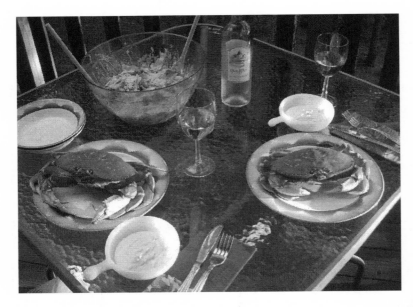

Dungeness crab, chilled or hot, with clarified butter or garlic aioli

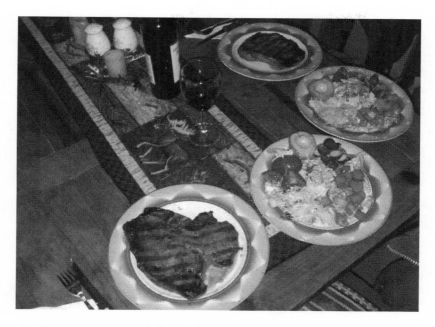

Grilled ribeye steaks and salad. Simple. Always works.

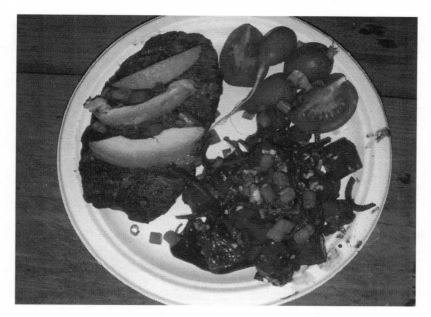

Grilled burger, watermelon tossed in reduced balsamic vinegar (yes, indeed), and other stuff for fun

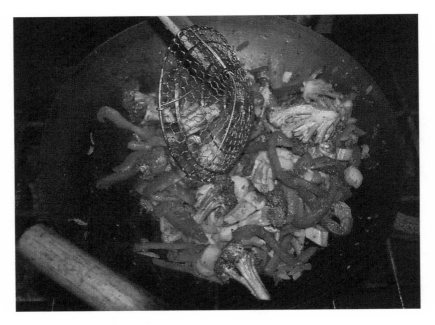

Wok grilled mixed vegetables, with coconut oil

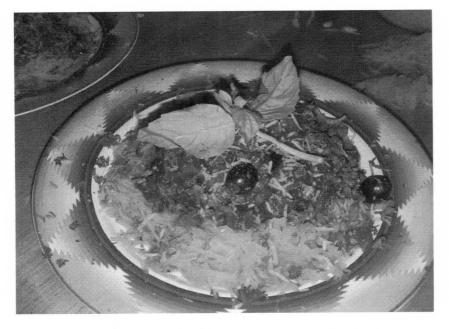

Spaghetti Squash with a meaty sauce. (Recipe)

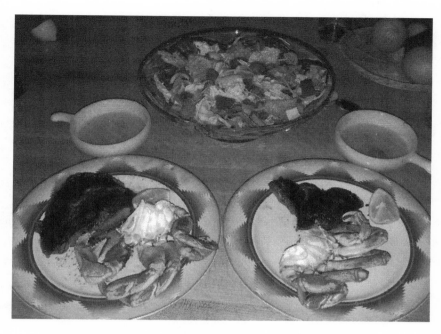

Classic surf & turf with a salad. All the stuff you love.

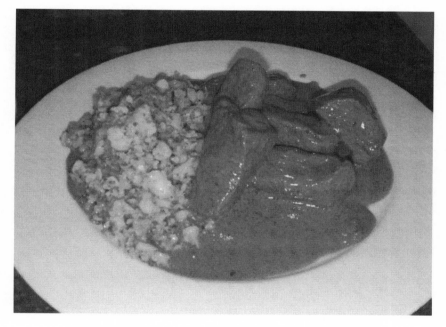

Steak tips and masaman curry sauce (Recipe)

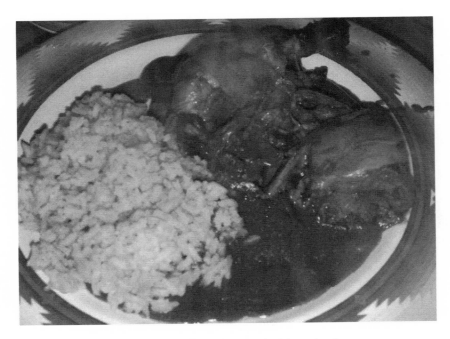

A unique "chicken mole" (Recipe)

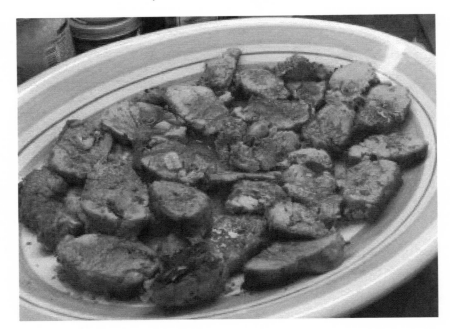

Stuff a pork loin with garlic cloves and rosemary. Toss it on the barbie. Do a spicy sauce.

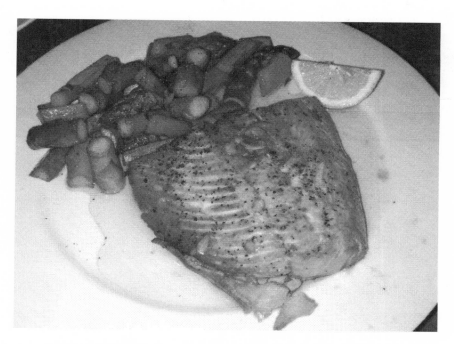

Basic grilled salmon and asparagus, butter and lemon

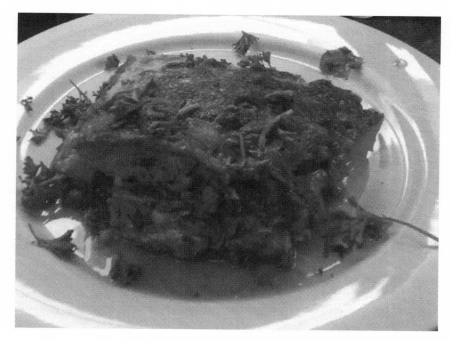

Missing lasagna? Then make it like Moussaka. (Recipe)

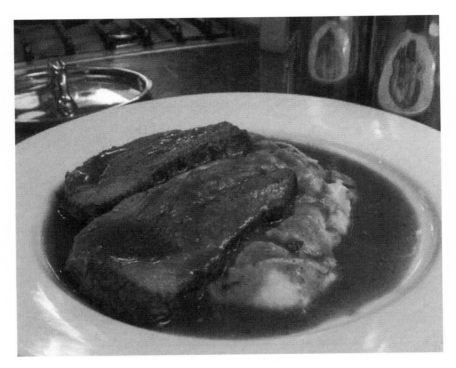

Basic grilled meat and potatoes, except with pureed celery root and a beef stock reduction.

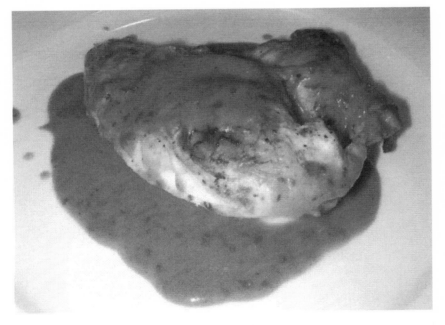

Grilled chicken, reducing chicken stock with butter and tarragon, where less is more.

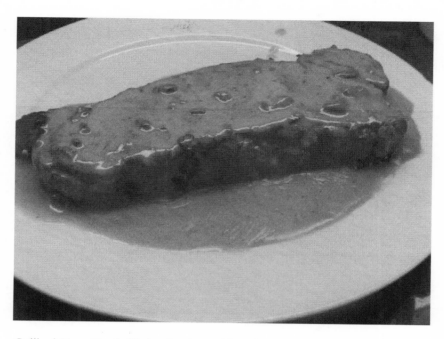

Grilled New York Strip. Reduced beef stock, butter, mushrooms

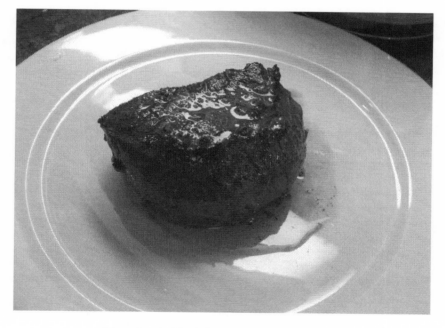

Simple. Grilled filet, browned butter.

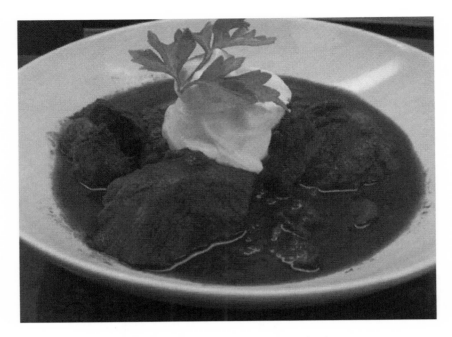

Texas Chili. No beans. (Recipe)

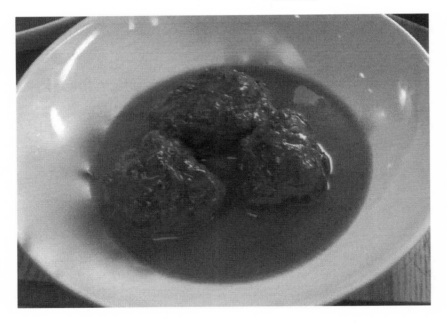

Meatballs in blue cheese sauce. (Recipe)

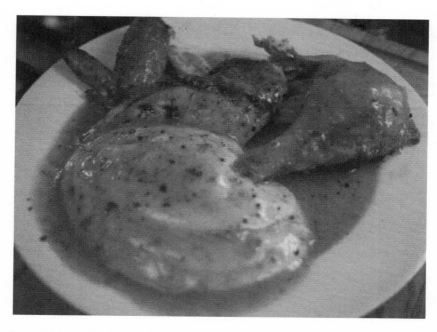

Comfort: Baked chicken and mashed potatoes & gravy. (Recipe)

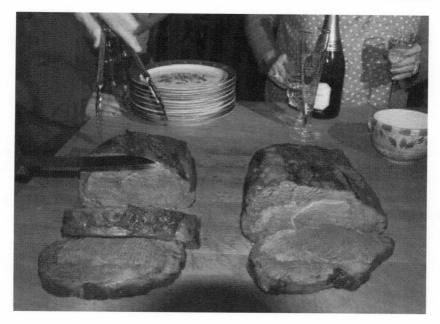

Prime Rib "Low & Slow" (200F until the meat is 125F internal, let it rest long)

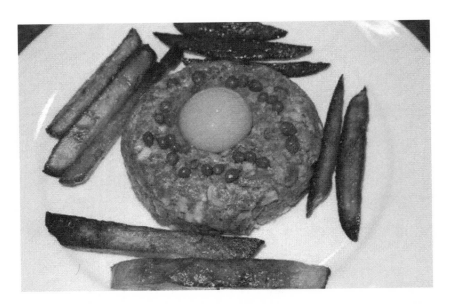

Are you hunter-gatherer enough? Steak Tartare. Chop it yourself. (Recipe)

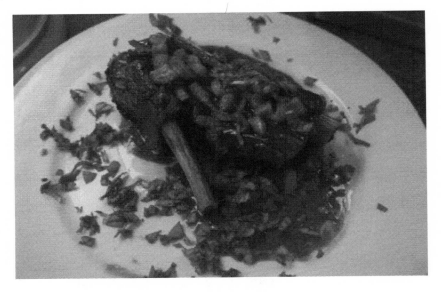

Braised beef short ribs and reduction and sauce

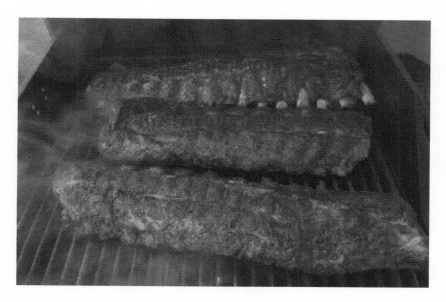

Dry rubbed baby back ribs and Paleo BBQ sauce. (Recipe)

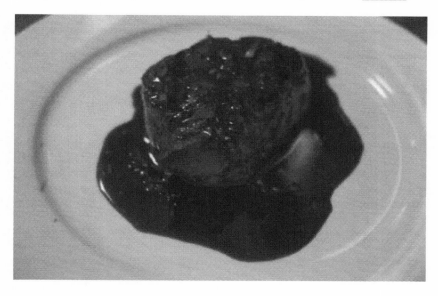

A grilled filet. Red wine sauce reduction to the equivalent of chocolate.

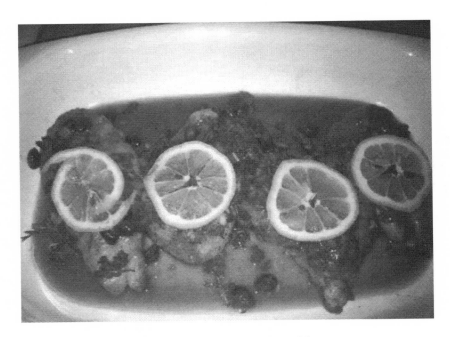

Chicken Picatta, Paleo fashion.

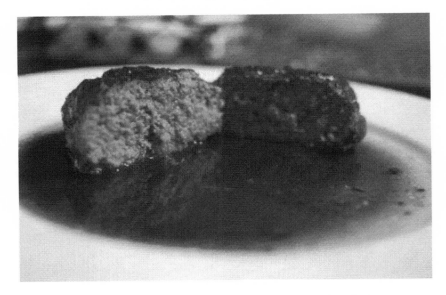

Burger done right, with a red wine reduction.

Appetizers

"Appetizers" in a Paleo sense can be a meal too. Or, it's meal you share with guests or even, a meal you save part of for the next day. Whatever the case, here's some ideas. I'm of the firm idea that appetizers are where you explore foods that are very highly nutritious, but that you may not be used to or, not wish to have in a meal sized portion.

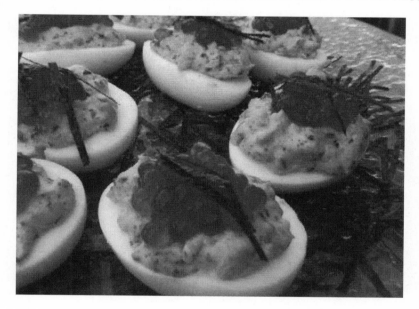

Deviled Eggs & Salmon Roe. (Recipe)

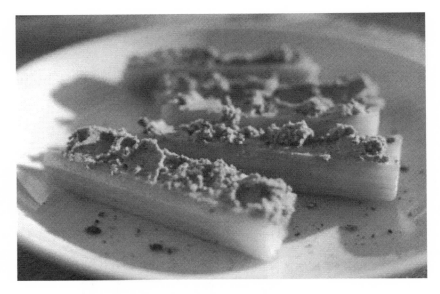

Beef and Chicken Liver Pate. (Recipe)

The Highest Nutrition

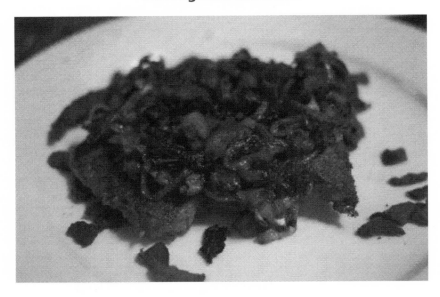

Liver and Onions. (Recipe)

Bread

There's only one proper recipe. This was a big effort getting right.

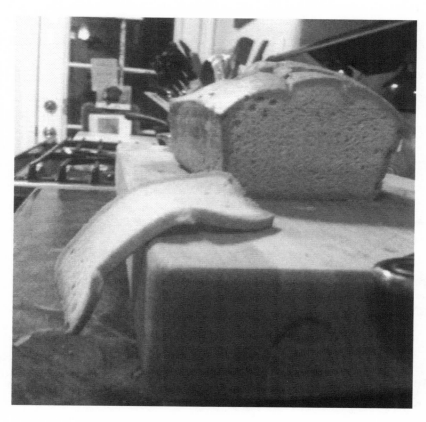

"Fat Bread." (Recipe)

All the foregoing things were those things I cooked at home. If you're trying to lose weight as I was, some years ago, did that represent *your* kitchen—what you were fixing at home? I'd guess not. Everyone is into convenience, now.

There's a single baked thing in all of that. It was the last thing and it took a lot of time, effort and experimentation to get it to a point where it's very unlikely to be a problem for anyone. A forthcoming cookbook will outline all the foregoing with detailed recipes, and many more.

Paleo Diet Recommended Supplements

People eating Paleo don't have to concern themselves with dietary supplements as much as do people on the SAD. We Paleo eaters are getting nutrients by way of eating nutritionally-dense food, which is the optimal way. There are, however, a few supplements that, owing to modern life and habits, are worthy of taking in as insurance:

1. Vitamin D

As previously discussed, Vitamin D protects you from cancer and a host of other diseases. Most people are severely deficient, and even more so the darker their skin and the father away from the equator. You should consider getting yourself tested. Aim for a level in the range of 50–80 ng/DL of 25 (OH)D, and adjust as necessary. Many blog readers find that it takes upwards of 5,000–10,000 IU per day of supplementation to get into that range and then, in combination with seasonal and sensible sun exposure, 4,000–6,000 IU per day year round to maintain it.

2. Omega-3 fatty acids

A natural, Paleolithic diet would have a ratio of omega-6 to omega-3 at anywhere from about .5/1 to 4/1. The typical American diet, with its high omega-6 vegetable oils, lies in a completely perverse range of 15/1 to 30/1. While a Paleo diet will bring you back into a normal ratio for a human animal, it's not a bad idea to hedge your bets and take a gram or two per day of fish oil or cod liver oil.

3. Vitamin K2, menatetrenone (MK-4)

K2 works to activate vitamins A and D, and helps to ensure that calcium and other minerals go everyplace they should (bones and teeth), and no place they shouldn't (arteries). The MK-4 subform is made by animals (from K1) for other animals (like us). It's interesting to note that the richest natural sources of MK-4 are to be found in eggs and mammalian milk (including human milk).

4. Magnesium

Our soil is now deficient beyond measure and vegetables aren't giving us a high enough amount of magnesium. Magnesium is a critical mineral implicated in over 300 cellular processes. While there are many different forms with differing absorption properties, I have had the best results with the 'Malate' formulation.

Additional Resources

- The Food Porn Category at Free the Animal with over 250 dishes with photos

- Free the Animal posts on Vitamin D

- Free The Animal posts on Vitamin K2

- Free the Animal posts on supplementation in general

Become a Hyperink reader. Get a special surprise.

Like the book? Support our author and leave a comment!

XV.

Success Stories

Paleo Diet Testimonials

One of the reasons I'm so enthusiastic about the Paleo way of life is that I've received thousands of emails and comments on my long-standing blog from people telling me all the ways in which they've improved their lives. They've lost substantial fat, ameliorated serious medical conditions . . . some people even tell me, "you saved my life." Ever had a bunch of people tell you that? I have, and seemingly out of the blue.

My grandmother, on the other hand, used to call me "the smart-ass." She was, in her 70s, a whiskey drinking cigarette smoker, so you know she had a twinkle in her eye when she said that. Yes, she was one of the loves of my life.

I enjoy both extremes on the spectrum of "terms of endearment." I can help save lives, and I'm definitely a smart-ass. I'm just some entrepreneurial guy who likes to take risks and likes to write, and who figured out a few things on his own.

But no matter what, my charge is this: *to be myself*.

What self are you? Are you hiding it? Does it scare you? Does it embarrass you? What are your results? And, how has it worked out for you?

Everyone with a non-sociopathic disposition wants to do well by themselves and others. As well, everyone with a non-sociopathic disposition is prone to influence from innumerable sources. Why do good people get fat and unattractive? Why don't we immediately recognize it as weird?

It's not just me. Thousands who suffered from obesity since childhood feel true confidence for the first time after starting the Paleo way. Men and women whose high weight and poor health prevented them from enjoying physical activity can now run, hike, climb, swim, and turn it up in bed.

Here's me somewhere along the way.

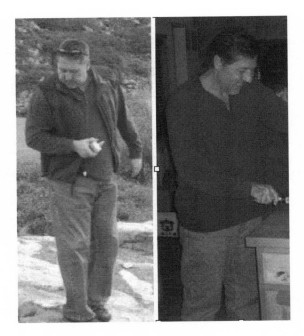

Same Shirt. Three years and 60 pounds later.

And my wife, Beatrice.

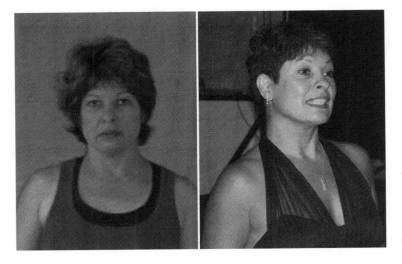

15 Months from picture-to-picture. The one on the right was her 50th birthday party.

While not my own success story, Super Mike nonetheless did himself well with an evolutionary approach to diet and exercise (he got his knowledge from Art De Vany).

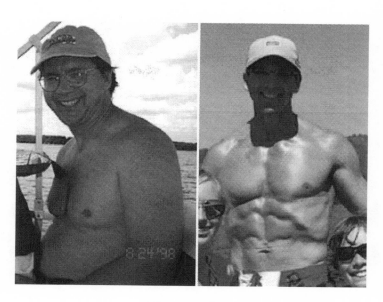

"Super Mike"

Tim went Paleo too.

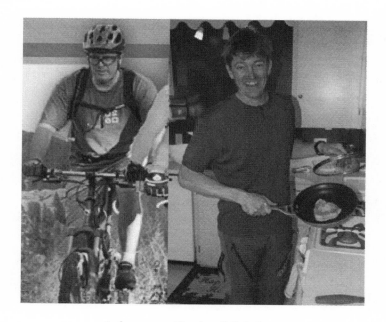

A few months is all it takes.

Murray downright Freed his Animal.

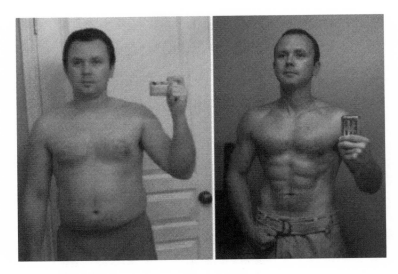

"I Freed My Animal."

"I just wanted to give you a quick message here to thank you for the awesome work you're doing with your website. I came across your site at the beginning of the year after seeing a link to your shampoo experiment, and really liked what I found. I had just started to try and get into shape (like I do for 2 weeks every January) using the old standby – 6 meals a day, whole grains, low fat, daily workouts, etc. I decided to try the caveman thing out, using your site (and Primal Blueprint, discovered as a link on your blog) as my sources of info.

"Well after about 6 months of doing this, which is 4 months longer than I've ever managed to keep to any kind of eating or fitness plan, I've lost 34 pounds and feel better than I have in years, going from 201 to 167. I'm surprised how easy this has been, with fat melting off me even at 36 years old. I'm in better shape than I was in my twenties.

"I'm also sending this now after reading your most recent post, maybe as another pat on the back to keep the great work up. There might be a rush of new bloggers coming out of the woodwork, but I'm sure I'd still be fat and cursing yet another failed New Year's Resolution if it wasn't for your blog.

"I'm attaching a couple of photos. The first is me at the end of 2009, and the second is a few days old, so basically 7 months between photos. I didn't do any measuring, have no idea what bodyfat is in either photo, all I know or care about is that I'm hauling around 34 less pounds of crap with me everywhere, and I feel better than ever.

"Thanks a million, man."

Timothy even got a writeup in Philadelphia Magazine.

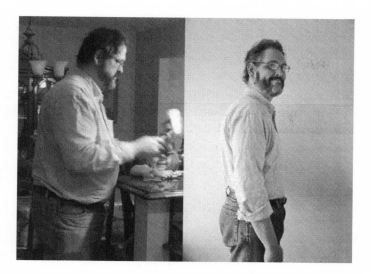

See? It's never too late.

Michelle from Australia is a Mark Sisson inspired transformation.

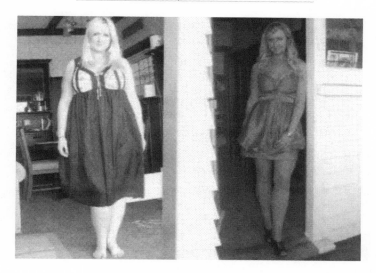

Women are animals too.

Austin from Singapore is a favorite of mine.

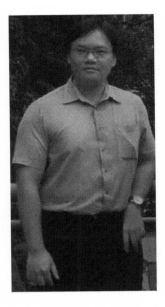

Oh, my. What shall he do?

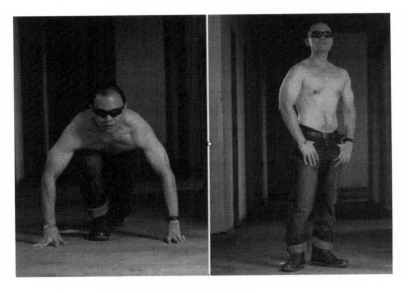

Of course. Go Paleo.

"I've been a reader of Free the Animal for over 6 months now, and enjoy it tremendously. I'll keep my story short. For the last 10 years, my weight has been hovering between 85 to 92kg, until concern over my long term health (my mother's family has a history of diabetes and hypertension) finally led me to to do something about my weight and eating habits in June of 2009. I'm currently 34 years old by the way.

"Google searches led me to Gary Taube's Good Calories Bad Calories, and blogs like Mark Sisson's Mark's Daily Apple, and Free the Animal. I applied what I learned, and slowly but steadily dropped nearly 20kg. My current weight is 70kg, and I went from size 34 jeans to size 30 jeans. The best thing is, I never, ever, felt hungry or deprived. I eat mostly real food,in the form of meat, vegetables & eggs, do IF occasionally, but I do eat a moderate amount of white rice daily. What can I say, I'm Chinese!

"Thanks Richard, for providing lots of useful information and entertainment throughout this process. I have to say It's a lot easier to identify with someone who is not a young stud and/or a former or current elite sportsman. I can't even begin to describe how my quality of life has improved since I made the change. Higher energy levels and no more dozing off in the office after lunch are just some of the things that come to mind. I'm in this for the long haul, and plan to continue to make progress in both health and body composition. As far as I'm concerned, there is always plenty of room for improvement."

Even an old gentleman like Chris can do it.

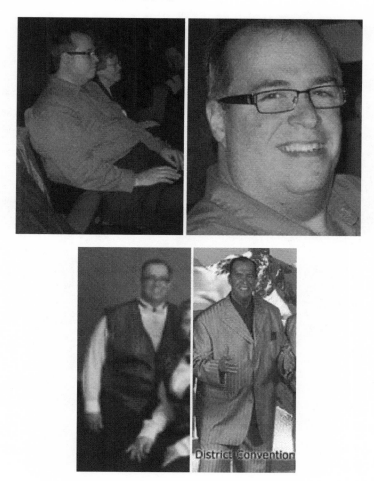

Music to my ears.

But can a vegan do herself better? Let's see.

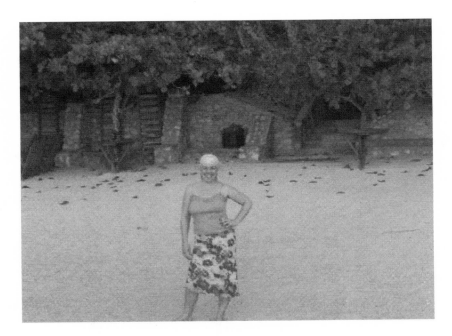

Vegan girl.

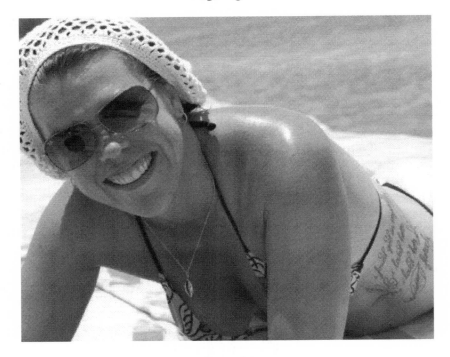

Cavegirl.

"Hi Richard,

"Long time reader....

"Mmmmm...veganism! it took me a while to learn the lesson that not eating meat is just a delusional quest for health.

"As a little girl, my very, very, very favorite food was filet mignon. My dad would actually chop it into tiny bites, deep fry it just so the outside was crisp and the inside was still blue and toss them to me like I was a little bird.

"At 18, I found idealism and became a vegetarian. I was one until I got pregnant with my son at 22. Those four years were the first time in my entire life that I struggled with weight. I just got thicker and thicker so just kept eliminating more and more fats and eating more and more grains in futility because that just led to me getting thicker and thicker. When I was in my first trimester, I started craving meat so badly that I ate it as much as I could (filled with guilt...those poor animals!) as raw as I could and eating grains at the other meals to pay for my sins.

"I omnivored it for the next 9 years. Then, I decided to go hardcore vegan. I never made it to the raw state and I can't even imagine the horror that my poor bowels would have had to go through if I had. As it was, I developed a horrible case of IBS with my seed oils, quinoa, and daily raw salad and tempeh salads. My depression reached an epic low (I did lose weight but I was not digesting a THING...it was literally going right through me). I did this for a year. I developed really painful eczema on my feet and hands and finally had to have surgery on my bowels. I have since discovered how gluten intolerant I am. I was also in constant pain. Sugar is vegan (well, brown sugar is...I wouldn't do white sugar because I'd read somewhere that bones were used to bleach it....honey was way off limits because the bees didn't make it for us... I was in a sad state!). My joints hurt, I was an insomniac. Truly it was ridiculous in hindsight....but, **I worked in a health food store and it was supposed to be such a health promoting diet that I just kept slogging through it. Possibly the worst side effect of my veganism was that I became such a self-righteous, pompous asswipe....**and I knew asswipes, what with the IBS and all. But I digress....

"One night at a party, my friend's husband, a chef, brought some pulled pork he'd smoked (I lived in the south) and I just fell into it as if it were a soft bed of delight. It wasn't until a year and a half ago that I found Mark's Daily Apple and then Free the Animal a little after that. I spent the entire summer doing it paleo. it **REVOLUTIONIZED** my life. My skin was beautiful again, I had energy to spare, My digestion was a thing of beauty....and I lost weight without trying.

"Last year, though, the earthquake hit Haiti, where I'm from, and when I went to help out the week after, I just had to eat whatever I could. When I was driving back from Miami, I was in a bad car accident that I'm only just NOW feeling mostly healed from. So, this past year has been very difficult because I've not been in a place to follow the lifestyle, as I haven't been in a position of controlling much of my food. BUT.....six weeks ago, I picked it all back up. I had wings for breakfast today after a fasted HIIT and lifting heavy things. Already in the past few weeks, I've debloated, sleep has been better, and energy is coming back in spades. YAY MEAT!

"Okay....that was a lot more than a meat story, but whatever.

"Thank you for your blog and your continued work!"

Here's one for the young guys who have the misfortune of starting the added fat process in college. here's Kit.

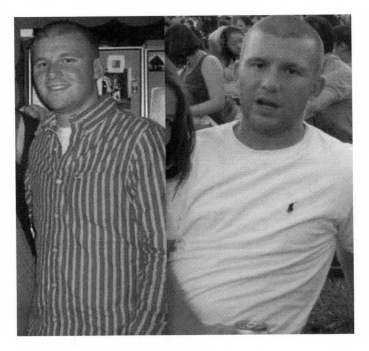

Big Kit.

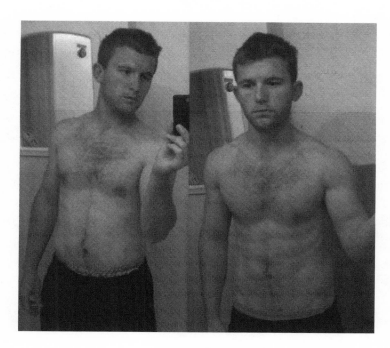

Less of Kit.

Mel, a PhD Biologist, emailed in from her med school research lab at a major university to tell me her success story. She lost 70 pounds and learned how to feed her kids healthy food. How lucky they are to be Paleo kids—they'll never have to undergo the toxic effects of SAD.

"I know you are a busy guy, so I will keep this e-mail to the point and try not to waste your time. I am another reader of your blog that appreciates your unorthodox approach to sharing insight about the paleo lifestyle. About six months ago I was first introduced to the low carb/paleo movement while reading Amy Alkon's blog. For most of my life I was never overweight, although I always had to closely watch how much I ate. However, after turning thirty and going through two pregnancies (I have a 9 month old and a 4 year old) I was seriously overweight and struggling with losing the excess pounds. It was getting to a point that I thought I might just be fat for the rest of my life — very depressing. However after reading Amy's posts on how eating meat and fat can actually help you lose weight, I immersed myself in the work of Gary Taubes

and Dr. Eades. In addition, I started doing my own literature searches about the effects of modern diet on metabolism. Much to my surprise (since this is not my field of research) these studies were more scientifically sound and made much more rational sense than any of the nutritional studies that we are normally told about through the media.

"After this research, it was not a hard decision to cut out all sugar, grains, and processed food from my diet. The results were spectacular. In a period of a little over six months, with very little effort (for example, I never went to the gym during this time — just hiked and played around with my kids), I was able to lose roughly 70 pounds and am now actually the weight that I was when playing competitive volleyball in college 15 years ago. Of course, this was all without ever going hungry and being able to eat delicious meals filled with lots of meat and buttered vegetables. In addition, this lifestyle is a great example for my kids since we all eat the same meals (versus mom eating a Lean Cuisine) and I now take them for a hike or we go to the park instead of me going to the gym to work out on the elliptical machine for hours at a time. I feel like I am setting them up to have a great relationship with food and their bodies for the rest of their lives.

"During this time I also started reading many of the paleo blogs. Your blog is one of my favorites because **my goal is not to live a "pure" paleo life full of "rules" that suck the fun out of everything**. I was already fat for 4 years and that was enough of a downer. I enjoy your blog because it is a breath of fresh air and full of vitality. **I don't want to be part of a cult** – I just want to be as healthy as I can possibly be and **not be told that I should feel guilty** because I sometimes eat (or feed my child) a potato! I get great ideas from your posts and enjoy your rants. You are not boring and you are**not dogmatic**. In my opinion, this is what makes your blog such a great read and source of information for people just starting to adopt this lifestyle.

"I am sure that you get tons of people thanking you for your blog, but I also wanted to add my thanks. I realize you don't get paid for doing this — so maybe knowing how much people appreciate your effort provides some reward. I have attached two pictures. The before picture is from June 2010 about a month after giving birth to my daughter. The second picture is from this morning."

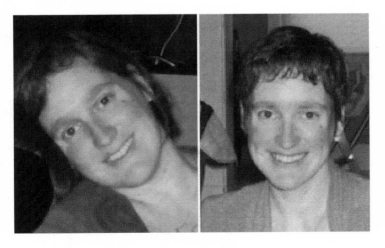

This is how I get paid the best.

Mike's just another "old guy." It's too late. Or, is it?

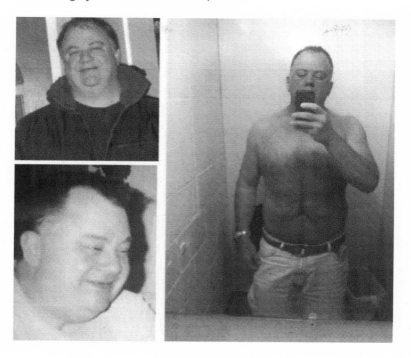

Life recapture.

And then there's Dan.

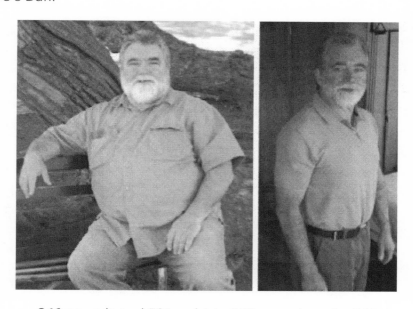

340 pounds and 52" waist to 183 pounds and a 34"

"The sudden death of my wife of 37 years prompted a lifestyle change that has led to a weight loss of 143 pounds in the last 20 months. After researching diet and nutrition. I've adopted a low carb/Paleo lifestyle.

"I tell my story on my blog at: http://danmoffett.blogspot.com/

Young guys too. Here's timothy.

"I love your blog. You reeled me in last year because, just like me, you were once a big fat slob who turned his life around on a dime via paleo. Your take-no-prisoners critiques of statism and other mass delusions are outstanding and make me want to jump out of my chair and hoist the black flag. You are the only blogger I know with these credentials and I have been fascinated and inspired by your prolific writing. Count me as a lifelong fan.

"I used to be a blithering idiot about health. Fast food every day, glued to CRTs and LCDs, my entire life an abuse of human heritage. Of course this caught up with me and I developed more health problems than I care to remember. It's a miracle I survived adolescence. Somehow I convinced the most beautiful woman I ever met to marry me when I was fat and broke and proceeded to drag her down with me.

"We finally conceived a child after years of adverse outcomes. Something inside me snapped then and I knew I had to fix myself. I started running everywhere and eating Subway. As I said, blithering idiot.

"Then I stumbled across Mark's Daily Apple. His concise writing style penetrated even my thick skull. Well, of course our bodies are designed to live as our ancestors did! How extremely stupid not to have thought of that. And I was an anthropology major. My glacial cognitive dissonance melted away overnight.

"I changed everything. How I ate, slept, trained, played, thought. My body responded instantly and I never looked back. I changed so drastically that I could no longer comprehend my former self. I resolved to make amends and build myself into a man that my distant ancestors would be proud of. This was in January 2010. I was 33 years old.

"I went from overweight to skinny. Then muscle started growing."

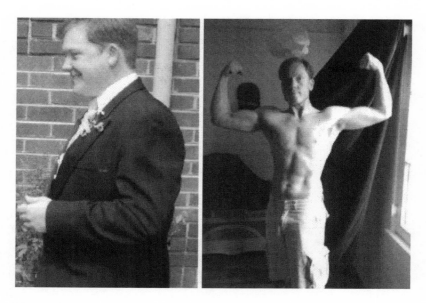

All based upon "bad and incomplete science." You be the judge.

Take Ricky, a reader of mine. A vegetarian for years, his diet consisted largely of pasta, cereals, fruit, and vegetables. In an effort to be healthy, he only consumed low-fat or skim milk. His blood pressure rose with his weight, which finally topped out at 262. That was when he lost his last bit of confidence.

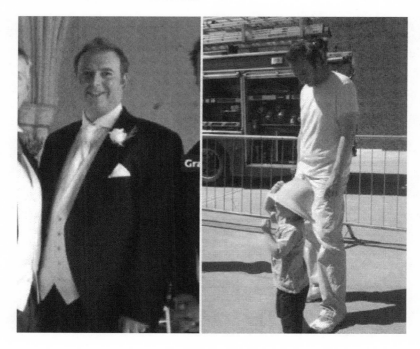

Ricky Graham

Browsing the Internet one day, he came upon an article about the "caveman diet."

Intrigued, he decided to give it a try—to learn how "bad" non-vegetarian food would make him feel. He started eating meat and fat, threw out the carbs, and walked a lot—at that point, he couldn't do much more.

But the weight started shedding from him. He lost 14 pounds each month for four months. He stopped weighing himself for awhile, as it was more about composition and energy for him at that point. At the one-year mark he decided to step on the scales: 173 pounds. In his words, *"A happy day, that one."*

I did an interview with Ricky from the UK, in three parts.

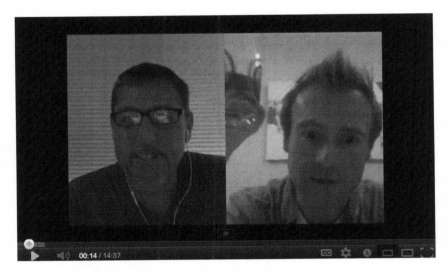

Part 1 / Part 2 / Part 3

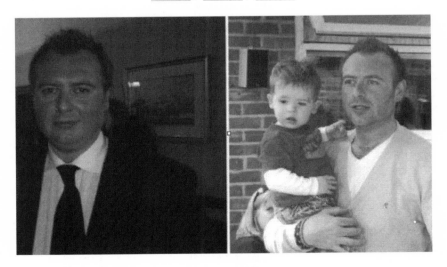

Can you imagine a motivation to get *your* health and body composition to normal? Ricky, I think found one.

Then there's the pair of parents who embraced the Paleo lifestyle with their three kids.

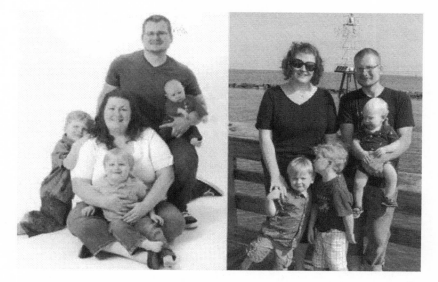

When Stacy and Matthew started living the lifestyle they experienced more than just fat loss—their family underwent a total health transformation, with improvements in depression, attention deficit disorder, and behavioral issues with their two older boys. You can read all about it here on their Paleo Parents blog.

I also did a video interview with Matt and Stacy.

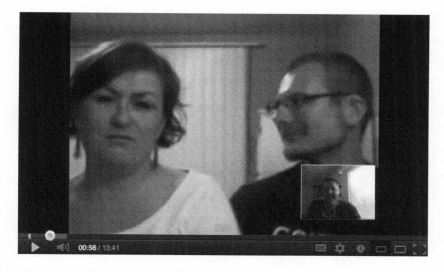

Part 1 / Part 2 *(about the children and behavioral issues—must watch)*

Back to the younger set, because it's all about humanity, rediscovering lost passion in life, for young and old alike.

Chris, for example.

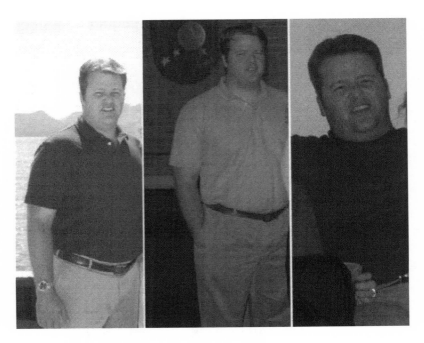

That's not going to work. What happens if I go Paleo?

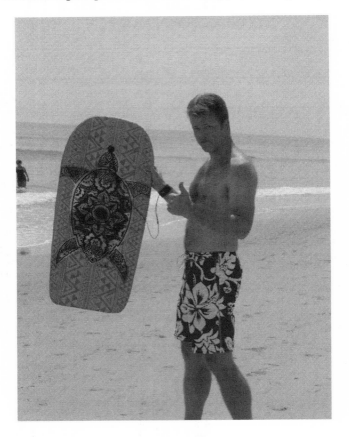

Show off.

I did a video interview with Chris as well.

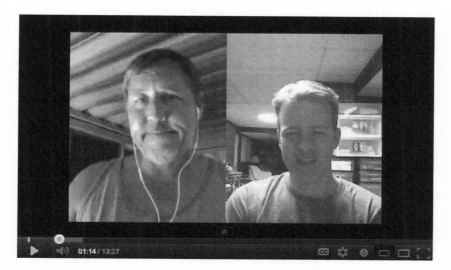

Watch here.

Timothy looks pretty damn happy to me. He got the love of his life to marry him when he was fat. But he decided to pay her back.

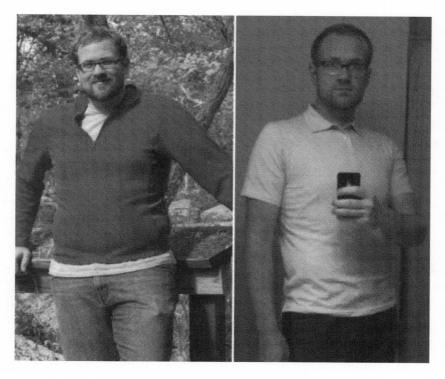

I'm sure she's happy about that.

Here's the interview where he tells the whole story.

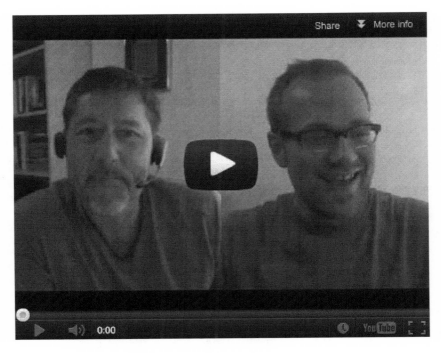

Watch the interview here.

I think this entire litany is something many men and women—young and old, scientifically educated or not—seem to be feeling, regretting, absolving, and all other sorts of emotions because in no way is it natural—ever—for a human animal to become fat and unattractive, relying upon social convention to keep a mate rather than earning it every day.

Every single day in this country and around the world, people are subjected to conventional "wisdom" and advice from the likes of Oprah, Dr. Oz, the medical and drug company establishment, the government-institution establishment, the industrial-agriculture food establishment, the talking heads in the media establishment, and health columnists. What kind of advice? Advice that keeps people in their 20s and 30s—and even children, in many cases—obese, immobile, grossly unattractive to the opposite sex, and sick. What's worse, it keeps them dependent on a system constructed for others' profit.

And isn't that what it's really all about, at the end of the day? The authorities don't want you using your own mind. They want nothing to do with your reasonable and rational self-experimentation on your own body. No, what they want is for you to recognize their "superior" intelligence and privileged access to information only they know how to properly interpret.

They want you to need them—to always look to them for your answers.

They want you to be skeptical—but only towards information that contradicts their diktats.

They want to be the authority, the last and final word—always and forever—and they aren't going to give that up without a fight.

Well, they've got themselves a fight.

Live Well

But will you make this *your* life's way?

What do *you* want?

What will *you* accept, and what will you settle for?

Taking account of your life to date, have some things gone wrong, and have some things gone right?

Being a relatively prosperous survivor in this wonder of life means—no, *guarantees*—that you not only did some things right, but that *you did a lot right*. So don't beat yourself up if your body doesn't look as it should, or your health is not where you'd like. If you follow the simple guidelines presented in this book, things will improve for you. Things can improve for the friends and family you care most about, too.

That's why this book was designed to be a quick read that almost anyone can get through quickly and understand. Anyone can literally begin right now.

So let's do a brief review.

Remember that above all, very little is being prescribed or proscribed here. These are ideas and suggestions as to how a human animal might best live in a modern society without giving up the advantages and conveniences beyond the awful food.

Secondly, there is no such thing as one diet for all. Our ancestors migrated to the far corners of the planet earth. They migrated to tropical regions, where they survived and thrived. They migrated to arctic regions, where they survived and thrived. Some occupied regions by seashores and lakes, some arid deserts, some mountain ranges upwards of 16,000 feet in elevation, and everything in between.

Throughout all these environments, a wide variety of plant and animal sources were used to sustain normal, human animal health. Where this wasn't possible, they had to move on to "greener pastures." Where it was, they gained *wisdom* over time, learning how best to exploit their natural environments to not only to survive, but to thrive optimally.

Don't buy into the notion—regardless of what you read elsewhere—that Paleo is zero-carb, low-carb, moderate-carb, high-protein, high-fat, low-fat, or anything of the kind.

The Paleo way is, simply, to eat a wide variety of real, whole, plant and animal sources in whatever combinations and ratios work best for you, determined over time and a bit of self experimenting. And what to avoid is equally straightforward: eat no grains or legumes, concentrated sugar, vegetable / seed oils . . . and figure out dairy for yourself. Avoid *all* processed foods in boxes, bags and freezer section,, and minimize eating out at restaurants.

Learn to become a competent and creative cook. Throw in a few of the recommended supplements to be on the safe side. Get your natural sunshine and sleep. Push, pull and lift some heavy things now and then. Run fast and go hungry sometimes. Engage in raucous sexual activity!

Eat well. Love well. Play well. *Live well.* I wish you all the best.

Become a Hyperink reader. Get a special surprise.

Like the book? Support our author and leave a comment!

XVI.

About The Blog

Free The Animal

You've seen references to my blog, Free the Animal throughout this e-book and I invite you to come visit and even join in the discussion if you like. Most posts get significant comments from readers, some newcomers and old hands that share of their own unique experiences in the Paleo lifestyle.

However, please understand that my blog is substantially different in style and use of language than that used in writing this book. In fact, my blog has been dubbed by some "the Paleo Pub." Accordingly, if you're offended by the frequent use of crude language, then don't say I didn't warn you.

Acknowledgements and Resources

Nobody really learns anything all on their own. Here are a few of the most important people and organizations I've learned from along the way. Most of the people involved have become friends of mine and have been very generous with their time.

Arthur De Vany, PhD

www.arthurdevany.com

Mark Sisson

www.marksdailyapple.com

Robb Wolf

robbwolf.com

Stephan Guyenet, PhD

wholehealthsource.org

Chris Masterjohn, PhD

www.cholesterol-and-health.com

Kurt Harris, MD

www.archevore.com

Michael Eades, MD

proteinpower.com

John Briffa, MD

www.drbriffa.com

Petro Dobromylskyj, DVM

high-fat-nutrition.blogspot.com

Anthony Colpo

anthonycolpo.com

Brad Pilon

eatstopeat.com

Erwan Le Corre

movnat.com

Martin Berkhan

www.leangains.com

Tom Naughton

www.fathead-movie.com

Weston A. Price Foundation

www.westonprice.org

Vitamin D Council

www.vitamindcouncil.org

GrassrootsHealthc

www.grassrootshealth.net

Become a Hyperink reader. Get a special surprise.

Like the book? Support our author and leave a comment!

About *The* Author

Richard Nikoley

Born & raised in Reno, Nevada. I attended and graduated from a small, religious-oriented private high school. Went on to attend a first year of college at a religious-oriented school in Chattanooga, Tennessee. I have had no interest in religious matters whatsoever for more than 25 years and don't plan on doing so again.

"Nothing in biology makes sense except in the light of evolution." - Theodosius Dobzhansky

I Graduated Oregon State University in 1984 with a bachelor's in Business Administration and two minor courses of study in mathematics / computer science, and naval science.

I was commissioned in the US Navy as a Surface Warfare Officer (SWO) immediately upon graduation from OSU. After some 8 months attending various schools in San Diego, CA, I traveled off to Yokosuka, Japan to join my first ship, the USS REEVES (CG-24), where I served from 1984-1987 as the Assistant Missiles Officer, First Lieutenant, and then finally, Electrical Officer.

After those first three years in Japan, I crossed the pier for another two years, joining the U.S. SEVENTH FLEET embarked aboard USS BLUE RIDGE (LCC-19). From 1988-1989 I was both the Assistant Fleet Scheduling Officer and the Assistant Logistics Officer. I managed a fuel budget of $180 million.

I left Japan after five years and headed to Monterey, California, where I was a student at the Defense Language Institute for the latter half of 1989. Upon successful completion of the French language course, I headed to Toulon, France, where from late 1989 - early 1992 I took up duties as an exchange officer with the French Navy: first aboard the FNS COLBERT (C 611), and later, the FNS DUQUESNE (D 603), both as the Navigator.

I left the US Navy in 1992 and returned to the U.S., San Francisco Bay Area. After a few false starts in entrepreneurial endeavors, I started a company in my bedroom in the summer of 1993 that evolved into what is today, Provanta Corp. I still regularly harass a modest cabal of employees.

Activity wise, I took up the sport of Hang-Gliding in 1996, and powered aircraft in 2005. Though I've soloed in the powered plane, I've yet to complete licensing requirements but plan to someday. I also fly sailplanes now and then.

In 2011 I celebrated my 10 year anniversary with my wife, Beatrice.

Book edited by **Theresa Noll.** *Theresa is a graduate of Oberlin College with seven years of editorial experience. Before moving to the Bay Area she rocked the New York publishing scene as managing editor of Seven Stories Press, where she worked with top thinkers such as Kurt Vonnegut, Howard Zinn, Russell Banks, Octavia Butler, and many more. She specializes in developmental editing and enjoys working closely with writers of all levels to help them reach their greatest potential.*

About the Publisher

Hyperink is the easiest way for anyone to publish a beautiful, high-quality book.

We work closely with subject matter experts to create each book. We cover topics ranging from higher education to job recruiting, from Android apps marketing to barefoot running.

If you have interesting knowledge that people are willing to pay for, especially if you've already produced content on the topic, please reach out to us! There's no writing required and it's a unique opportunity to build your own brand and earn royalties.

Hyperink is based in SF and actively hiring people who want to shape publishing's future. Email us if you'd like to meet our team!

Note: If you're reading this book in print or on a device that's not web-enabled, **please email** books@hyperinkpress.com with the title of this book in the subject line. We'll send you a PDF copy, so you can access all of the great content we've included as clickable links.

Get in touch: 🐦 f ✉

Other Awesome Books

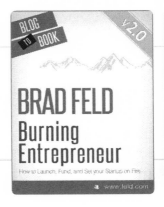
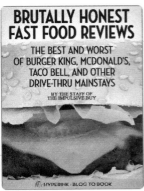
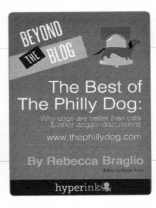
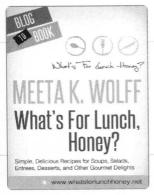

Hyperink Benefits

★ Interesting Insights ★ The Best Commentary ★ Shocking Trivia

- Business School For Startups

- Notes from the Startup Wilderness: Discovery Engines, Big Data Mining,...

- Sacha Greif's Thinking Like A Designer

- Brutally Honest Fast Food Reviews: The Best and Worst of Burger King,...

- Philly Dog: Why Dogs are Better Than Cats

- The Startup Law Playbook

- My Itchy Travel Feet: Breathtaking Adventure Vacation Ideas

- Rock Star Productivity: Time Management Tips, Leadership Skills, and Other...

- ...

- What's For Lunch, Honey?

37233284R00106